Statistics for Nurses

Statistics for Nurses

EVELYN CAULCOTT MA

Senior Lecturer
Department of Social Science and Administration
Goldsmiths' College, University of London

SCUTARI PRESS London

Published by Scutari Press, a division of Scutari Projects Ltd, the publishing company of the Royal College of Nursing, London

First published 1992

Reprinted 1994

British Library Cataloguing-in-Publication Data

Caulcott, Evelyn.
  Statistics for nurses.
  I.Title
  001.4

  ISBN 1-871364-71-X

Typeset by Blackpool Typesetting Services Ltd, Blackpool
Printed by Page Bros, Norwich

For Celia
and in memory of Stephen

Contents

Preface

This book is intended as a basic text for students in training for the Registered General Nurse qualification, primarily for those who are nursing degree students, but also for other students, particularly in the health field, who find themselves in need of a basic text on statistics. It is further intended for postgraduate students and nurses already qualified who seek guidance on statistics and statistical techniques, especially in relation to research. Statistical methods are the same, irrespective of their context, but for intended users, a textbook directed to their field is more helpful than a statistics textbook of a general kind, or one written for users in another field.

The aim is to provide a reference text for those handling and interpreting data, or engaged in research. It is also a tool for those who have to conduct statistical computations, and examples of calculations are included. The nature of measures and their use is discussed so that the reader can select appropriate techniques.

No assumptions are made about the mathematical capacities of readers, other than an ability to operate the four rules of arithmetic (that is, to be able to add, subtract, multiply and divide), and to use a calculator to assist in these activities. The Mathematical Note (p. xvii) provides aid for those whose mathematical qualifications are limited or lapsed. Other necessary underpinnings such as the calculation of percentages, ratios, use of graphs and the interpretation and use of algebraic formulae, are covered in the text. The Glossary of Symbols and Formulae (p. xxi), on a chapter by chapter basis, provides an additional reference source.

Statistics is an entirely logical subject. There are two very valuable qualities to be cultivated when operating in the field of statistics. The first might be called a crude sense of the quantitative—are orders of magnitude right? What are the implications? Where should emphasis lie? The second is informed commonsense—do figures look sensible? Do they fit into logical patterns? Are there unexpected peculiarities? If so, can they be accounted for? Statistics and statistical methods are tools to be put to good use, with an awareness of their benefits and limitations.

Acknowledgements

I am grateful to the following sources for permission to publish data in tables in the text:

Tables 2.1, 2.2, 4.1 and 5.3 from DH (1989). *Health and Personal Social Service Statistics for England 1989*, HMSO.
Table 3.1 from CSO (1988). *Social Trends 18 1988*, HMSO.
Table 4.4 from CSO (1990). *Social Trends 20 1990*, HMSO.
Tables 4.2 and 13.4 (adapted) from OPCS (1989). *General Household Survey 1987*, HMSO.
Table 15.3 from OPCS (1975, 1981, 1986, 1990). *Population Trends 1, 26, 46, 62*, HMSO.

The material from government publications is reproduced with the permission of the Controller of HMSO.

I am grateful to the Statistics and Research Division of the Department of Health for providing me with the data on age of hospital dental staff, 1987 from which the samples in chapter eight were drawn.

I am indebted to the *Biometrika* Trustees for permission to reproduce material taken from Tables 1 and 18 of the *Biometrika Tables for Statisticians* Vol 1 (3rd Edition, 1966) edited by E S Pearson and H O Hartley.

I am grateful to the Literary Executor of the late Sir Ronald A Fisher, FRS to Dr Frank Yates, FRS and the Longman Group Ltd, London for permission to reprint Tables III and IV from their book *Statistical Tables for Biological, Agricultural and Medical Research* (6th edition, 1974).

I appreciate the permission from Collins English Dictionaries of Harper Collins Publishers to use the definitions included in chapter seven which are taken from Collins English Dictionary (3rd Edition, 1991).

I would like to express appreciation of the support of Anne Betts of the Institute of Advanced Nursing Education of the Royal College of Nursing who was instrumental in my writing this book. I am indebted to her, and to other readers from the nursing profession, for advice and comments which have proved invaluable.

I am grateful to my friend and colleague Myra Woolf for her helpful comments particularly on chapter nine, to the resources and staff of the Computer Centre at Goldsmiths' College, and to my editor Patrick West for his support.

Mathematical Note:
A Reminder for the Uncertain

Our tools are the four rules of arithmetic—we must be able to add, subtract, multiply and divide, aided by a pocket calculator.* We need to remember the operational rules about the sequence of steps in a computation. Here is your guide:

1. multiplying and dividing take precedence over adding and subtracting.
2. brackets are worked out first;
3. a dividing (fraction) line acts as a bracket;
4. a square root expression also behaves as a bracket;
5. a power sign—a squared number—outside a bracket affects everything in the bracket.

An example:

$$63 + \frac{47 - 25}{17} \times 12$$

is processed as follows.

1. The dividing line acts as a bracket, so complete the subtraction [47 − 25] to get 22,

$$63 + \frac{22}{17} \times 12$$

2. now divide 22 by 17, and multiply the result by 12 (it would not matter if we had multiplied 22 by 12 and then divided the product by 17; the outcome is the same),[†]

$$63 + 1.2941 \times 12$$
$$= 63 + 15.5292$$
$$= 78.5292$$

---

* A simple basic calculator costing a few pounds is required. It should have a memory in which numbers can be accumulated, a square root facility and a percentage facility. More elaborate, and hence more expensive calculators, may not help much more than a basic calculator, and their operation may be more complicated.

† There is a marginal difference between the alternative calculations in the fourth place of decimals because of the rounding of the result of 22 ÷ 17. This discrepancy disappears when rounding the final answer to 2 places of decimals.

$$\text{OR} \quad 63 + \frac{264}{17}$$

$$= 63 + 15.5294$$

$$= 78.5294$$

3. finally round the answer to 2 places of decimals

$$= 78.53$$

Another example:

$$\sqrt{\frac{1,747}{23} - \left(\frac{19}{6}\right)^2}$$

1. Work out the two divisions, $1,747 \div 23$ and $19 \div 6$;

$$\sqrt{75.9565 - (3.1667)^2}$$

2. now square 3.1667 (multiply it by itself);

$$\sqrt{75.9565 - 10.0280*}$$

[* We would get the same result if we had squared 19 getting 361, squared 6 getting 36 and then divided 361 by 36.]

3. complete the subtraction, now only requiring the square root;

$$\sqrt{65.9285}$$

4. obtain the square root;

$$8.1196$$

5. finally round the answer to 2 places of decimals;

$$8.12$$

These are two useful examples of the sort of calculation we shall come across later. So remember to look back at this section.

Accuracy

How accurate should we be in our calculations? There are two issues:

1. accuracy in the *process* of calculation;
2. accuracy of the final *result*.

We must be *more* accurate during the process of calculation than the accuracy required in the final answer. A good rule of thumb is that the accuracy during the process of calculation should be to 2 significant figures more than we expect to require of the answer. For example, if we wish to

obtain bed-occupancy rates to 1 place of decimals, the body of the calculation should be conducted to 3 places of decimals. The final answer is
rounded to 1 place of decimals. This degree of accuracy in the process of
calculation is a protection against error. By their nature some calculations
easily produce incorrect answers if any material rounding is introduced in
the process of calculation.

Using a calculator efficiently eliminates this problem. The eight significant figure operation of the standard pocket calculator provides adequate
accuracy. To benefit from this, the calculation should as far as possible be
carried out in the calculator itself (with suitable noting of key figures). The
memory of the calculator is used to 'store' stages during the process of
computation. This avoids the reentering of numbers for successive steps—
always a source of error. The following reworking of the second example
above demonstrates the use of the calculator memory.

$$\sqrt{\frac{1,747}{23} - \left(\frac{19}{6}\right)^2}$$

With the calculator:
1. enter $1747 \div 23$
   display   75.956521
2. enter display into memory (M+)
3. enter $19 \div 6$
   display   3.1666666
4. enter square
   [see calculator instructions; either a square key (x^2) or simply press
   $\times$ (multiply) then the = key after the number you wish to square is
   on the display]
5. display   10.027777
6. enter display into memory to *subtract* (M−)
7. enter memory recall   (MR)
8. display   65.928744
9. enter square root   ($\sqrt{}$)
10. display   8.1196517
11. round answer   8.12

The accuracy we require in the final result depends on the general magnitude of the data, its level of accuracy and, how precise an answer we need
having regard to the purposes for which it is to be used. A subjective
decision. If we must err, we should do so in the direction of being rather
more accurate than we might finally require, rather than risk an insufficiently accurate or too rounded a result. Some of the results of computations
in this text are presented at a higher degree of accuracy than is strictly
necessary or justified by the data. The final step is to round the results
appropriately.

Glossary of Symbols and Formulae

Chapter 5

$\bar{x}$ (pronounced x-bar) arithmetic mean of a variable; used for sample data.

x_i (pronounced x-i) representative value of a variable x.

n total number of items, sample size.

Σ (pronounced sigma) Greek (capital) letter used to indicate the items following are summed.

$\displaystyle\sum_{i=1}^{n} x_i$ $= x_1 + x_2 + x_3 + x_4 + \cdots + x_n$.

Subscripts indicate different values of x. The limits to $\sum x_i$ $(i = 1, n)$ indicate the range of values to be summed, x_i from $i = 1$ to n.

$\dfrac{\sum x}{n}$ mean of ungrouped data.

f frequency, of a variable value.

xf value x of a variable multiplied by frequency f, the number of times x occurs.

$\dfrac{\sum xf}{n}$ mean of grouped data.

$L_m + \dfrac{B_m \times C_m}{F_m}$ median (see text for notation definitions).

Chapter 6

s standard deviation, of a sample.

$\sqrt{\dfrac{\sum (x - \bar{x})^2}{n}}$ standard deviation, definitional formula.

$\sqrt{\dfrac{\sum x^2}{n} - \left(\dfrac{\sum x}{n}\right)^2}$ standard deviation, ungrouped data.

$x^2 f$ — value of variable x, squared and multiplied by f, the frequency with which x occurs. Note that f is *not* squared.

$$\sqrt{\frac{\sum x^2 f}{n} - \left(\frac{\sum xf}{n}\right)^2}$$ — standard deviation, grouped data.

$\frac{s}{\bar{x}} \times 100$ — coefficient of variation.

s^2 — variance.

Chapter 7

μ (pronounced mew) — Greek letter representing the population mean.

σ (pronounced sigma) — Greek (lower case) letter representing the population standard deviation.

p — the probability of an event occurring.

$1 - p$ — the probability of an event not occurring where p is the probability of the event occurring.

$[p + (1 - p)]^n$ — form of the binomial distribution used in probability situations; p is the probability of 'success', $(1 - p)$ the probability of 'failure', and n is the number of trials.

np — mean of binomial distribution.

$\sqrt{np(1 - p)}$ — standard deviation of binomial distribution.

standard normal distribution — a normal distribution with mean of 0, standard deviation of 1, and total area under the curve equal to 1.

$z = \dfrac{x - \mu}{\sigma}$ — standard units value, or z-value, of x, where μ is the mean and σ the standard deviation of the distribution from which x is drawn.

Chapter 8

$\sigma/\sqrt{n}$ — standard deviation of theoretical sampling distribution, a normal distribution, of means of samples size n, when drawn from a population with standard deviation σ.

θ (pronounced theta) — Greek letter used to indicate a population proportion/percentage.

$\theta\%$

mean percentage of a binomial distribution expressed in percentages.

$\sqrt{\dfrac{\theta\%(100 - \theta)\%}{n}}$

standard deviation of a binomial distribution expressed in percentages. Also standard deviation of theoretical sampling distribution of percentages of samples, size n, when drawn from a population itself having a percentage θ.

Chapter 10

confidence limits

range of values within which, with a stated probability, a population parameter is expected to fall.

standard error

standard deviation of a sampling distribution.

$se_{\bar{x}}$

standard error of the mean.

$se_{\bar{x}}$

$= \sigma/\sqrt{n}$ if the population standard deviation is known, or $s/\sqrt{n}$ if the sample standard deviation is being used as 'best estimate' of the population standard deviation.

N

number of units in population.

$\sqrt{\dfrac{N - n}{N - 1}}$

small population correction.

t distribution

theoretical distribution to which distributions of means of small samples approximate.

t

statistic equivalent to a z-value for samples size 30 or less.

se_p

standard error of the proportion or percentage.

se_p

$= \sqrt{\dfrac{p(1 - p)}{n}}$ or $\sqrt{\dfrac{p\%(100 - p)\%}{n}}$

Chapter 11

$z = \dfrac{\bar{x} - \mu}{se_{\bar{x}}}$

standard units value (large sample) for difference between sample and population means.

$|\ |$

indicates that the sign (+ or −) of the number or symbol between the upright parallel lines is to be ignored.

$>$

greater than the expression or value following.

$<$

less than the expression or value following.

$z_{0.05}$

z-value corresponding to 0.05 probability which excludes 0.05 (5%) of the total area under a normal curve, outside the values $-z_{0.05}$ to $+z_{0.05}$.

$z_{0.01}, z_{0.001}$ — other subscripts refer similarly to other probabilities.

$t = \dfrac{\bar{x} - \mu}{se_{\bar{x}}}$ — t-value (small samples), comparable to a z-value where the sample size is 30 or less.

$t_{0.05}, t_{0.01}, t_{0.001}$ — values of t corresponding to probabilities 0.05, 0.01 and 0.001.

Chapter 12

μ_1, μ_2 — means of different populations, distinguished by subscript.

σ_1, σ_2 — standard deviations of populations with means μ_1 and μ_2.

n_1, n_2 — sizes of samples drawn from populations with means μ_1 and μ_2.

s_1, s_2 — standard deviations of samples with means $\bar{x}_1$ and $\bar{x}_2$.

$se_{\bar{x}_1 - \bar{x}_2}$ — the standard error of the difference between two sample means, $(\bar{x}_1 - \bar{x}_2)$.

$se_{\bar{x}_1 - \bar{x}_2}$ — $= \sqrt{\dfrac{\sigma_1^2}{n_1} + \dfrac{\sigma_2^2}{n_2}}$ if the population standard deviations are known, or $\sqrt{\dfrac{s_1^2}{n_1} + \dfrac{s_2^2}{n_2}}$ if the sample standard deviations are being used as 'best estimates' of the corresponding population standard deviations.

$\geq$ — greater than or equal to the expression or value following.

$z = \dfrac{\bar{x}_1 - \bar{x}_2}{se_{\bar{x}_1 - \bar{x}_2}}$ — standard units value for the difference between two sample means (large samples).

$t = \dfrac{\bar{x}_1 - \bar{x}_2}{se_{\bar{x}_1 - \bar{x}_2}}$ — standard units value for the difference between two sample means (small samples).

$se_{\bar{x}_1 - \bar{x}_2}$ (small samples) — $= \sqrt{\dfrac{(n_1 - 1)s_1^2 + (n_2 - 1)s_2^2}{(n_1 - 1) + (n_2 - 1)} \left(\dfrac{1}{n_1} + \dfrac{1}{n_2} \right)}.$

$\theta_1\%, \theta_2\%$ — percentages in two separate populations.

$p_1\%, p_2\%$ — percentages in single samples drawn from populations with percentages $\theta_1\%$ and $\theta_2\%$.

$se_{p_1 - p_2}$ — standard error of the difference between two sample percentages, $(p_1\% - p_2\%)$.

$se_{p_1-p_2}$ $= \sqrt{\dfrac{\theta_1\%(100 - \theta_1)\%}{n_1} + \dfrac{\theta_2\%(100 - \theta_2)\%}{n_2}}$

where the samples are drawn from two separate populations whose percentages are known, or

$\sqrt{\dfrac{p_1\%(100 - p_1)\%}{n_1} + \dfrac{p_2\%(100 - p_2)\%}{n_2}}$

where the sample percentages are being used as 'best estimates' of the unknown population percentages, $\theta_1\%$ and $\theta_2\%$.

$z = \dfrac{p_1 - p_2}{se_{p_1-p_2}}$ standard units value for the difference between two sample percentages.

Chapter 13

χ (pronounced ki)   Greek letter (chi) used to represent a multinomial distribution.

o_i general representation of observed value.

e_i general representation of expected value, corresponding to observed value, o_i.

χ^2 (chi-square)   statistic computed for the chi-square test.

χ^2 $= \sum \dfrac{(o - e)^2}{e}$

r number of rows in a contingency table.

k number of columns in a contingency table.

$(r - 1) \times (k - 1)$ number of degrees of freedom in an $r \times k$ contingency table.

$\chi^2_{0.05}, \chi^2_{0.01}, \chi^2_{0.001}$ values of χ^2 corresponding to probabilities 0.05, 0.01 and 0.001.

C contingency coefficient.

C $= \sqrt{\dfrac{\chi^2}{\chi^2 + N}}$

N total of all samples included in contingency table.

Chapter 14

F a theoretical distribution.

F $= \dfrac{\sum s_b^2}{\sum s_w^2}.$

s_b^2 variance between sample means.

s_b^2

$$= \frac{n[\sum x_i^2 - \{(\sum x_i)^2/k\}]}{k - 1} \text{ where } k \text{ is the number}$$

of samples each of size n, and x_i is the representative value of the sample means, or

$$\frac{\sum x_i^2 n_i - [(\sum x_i n_i)^2/N]}{k - 1} \text{ where } x_i \text{ is the repre-}$$

sentative value of means of k unequal samples size n_i. Total sample size is N where $N = \sum n_i$.

s_w^2 variance within samples.

s_w^2

$$= \frac{\sum s_i^2}{k} \text{ where } s_i^2 \text{ is the representative variance of}$$

k equal sized samples, or $\dfrac{\sum (n_i - 1)s_i^2}{N - k}$ for k

unequal sized samples, with n_i the representative sample size.

$F_{0.05}, F_{0.01}$ values of F corresponding to probabilities 0.05 and 0.01.

Chapter 15

y value of dependent variable.

x value of independent variable.

$y = a + bx$ general equation of a straight line used for regression line.

a, b regression coefficients.

a intercept on y-axis when $x = 0$.

b slope or gradient of line.

scatter diagram   graph in which values of x are plotted along the horizontal axis, paired with values of y which are plotted along the vertical axis.

b

$$= \frac{n \sum x_i y_i - \sum x_i \sum y_i}{n \sum x_i^2 - (\sum x_i)^2}$$

a

$$= \frac{\sum y_i - b \sum x_i}{n} \text{ where } x_i, y_i \text{ are representative}$$

values of the independent variable x and the dependent variable y, and n is the number of pairs of values of x and y.

$y = a + b_1 x_1 + b_2 x_2 + b_3 x_3$ multiple regression equation with independent variables x_1, x_2, x_3.

Chapter 16

r

correlation coefficient, referred to also as the product moment correlation coefficient.

r

$$= \sqrt{\frac{\text{explained variance}}{\text{total variance}}}$$

$$= \frac{n \sum x_i y_i - \sum x_i \sum y_i}{\sqrt{[n \sum x_i^2 - (\sum x_i)^2][n \sum y_i^2 - (\sum y_i)^2]}}$$

se_r

standard error of the correlation coefficient, r.

se_r

$= 1/\sqrt{n-2}$ on the assumption that the true correlation is zero, or $\dfrac{1-r^2}{n-2}$ for any given value of r, and which can therefore be used to derive confidence limits for r.

$z = \dfrac{r}{se_r}$

standard units value for the difference between the calculated value of r and $r = 0$, used when testing the null hypothesis that there is no association between the variables x and y.

coefficient of determination

$= r^2 \times 100$

r'

rank correlation coefficient.

r'

$= 1 - \dfrac{6 \sum d_i^2}{n(n^2 - 1)}$ where d_i is the difference between

the ranks of paired values, x_i and y_i.

1

Introduction

The term 'statistics' can mean different things in different contexts. Firstly, it can refer to simple numerical data, the raw material which is presented in tables or graphically. At this level, definition, accuracy, reliability and comparability of data, aspects related to the counting process, are extremely important.

Secondly, 'statistics' can refer to measures calculated from basic data, such as arithmetic mean or median, which describe the data in some way. This is an extension of the information provided by the raw data itself.

Thirdly, statistics can be inferential. Data can be examined against theoretical criteria which permit inference about the patterns shown by the data. Statistical tests can establish differences between groups. Inferential statistics contribute by indicating a real change, a real difference. If this statistical evidence did not exist, it would be pointless to pursue questions of cause and effect—why groups were different. The inferential evidence is a necessary contribution and an invaluable starting point.

Finally, there are techniques of statistical analysis which are a means of examining data to see the relationship between different sources of information. Again, establishing a statistical association between variables is a necessary preliminary to consideration of cause and effect but this can only be confirmed through evidence from other sources.

This book covers these different facets of statistics. Part I deals with aspects of collecting, classifying and presenting data in tables and graphically. It also covers interpreting data shown in tables. These are very basic aspects of using statistics. Part II extends to simple descriptive measures, mean, standard deviation, median and the quantiles and the cirumstances in which these are used. Parts I and II are concerned with presentation of statistical data in informative ways.

Part III deals with sample data, the source material of inferential statistics. Starting with an account of sampling theory and the relationship between sampling and research designs, it proceeds to estimation of population parameters from sample statistics, and to tests concerning differences between sample means or percentages. The techniques discussed are essential to those concerned with research.

Finally, Part IV looks at two variables in terms of the relationship which can be established between them, and the strength of that relationship. This is an introduction to an important and complex area of statistical analysis, the fundamental principles of which are discussed here.

Each chapter has suggestions for further reading, together with examples for the reader's own practice. The Mathematical Note (p. xvii) provides a reminder of simple computation using a calculator. The Glossary of Symbols and Formulae (p. xxi) is a convenient summary and can be used to identify the chapter in which a particular formula is discussed.

The calculations carried out in the text assume the use of a calculator. The emphasis on methods of computation contributes to an understanding of how the data is handled, how the result relates to the data and what can be inferred from the result. Some more complex calculators, often referred to as 'scientific', are programmed to carry out computations (such as mean, standard deviation, regression coefficients, correlation coefficient). These programmes are designed for original (ungrouped) data and are suitable for small quantities of data only. Additionally, such calculators do not provide a record of the data entered, so there is no easy means of checking this (a problem which does not arise with computers). There are risks of error, and computations must be repeated at least twice, preferably by different persons, to ensure correctness. It is safer to use a computer which will provide a record both of data entered, and the computations carried out.

The use of computers is not covered although reference is made to the way in which data is handled logically by computers. For those handling large quantities of data, or involved in research with more than a very modest number of cases, and seeking to use inferential and analytical techniques, there are good software packages available for computer analysis. Explore the software locally available.

Introductory Reading

For a light-hearted introduction to statistics:

Huff D (1973) *How to Lie with Statistics*. London: Penguin.

More demanding, but worth exploring:

Bartholomew D J and Bassett E E (1971) *Let's Look at the Figures*. London: Penguin.
Meek R L (1971) *Figuring out Society*. London: Fontana/Collins.
[Try Chapter 1]

Part I

Basic Data

2

Collecting, Classifying and Presenting Data

2.1 Collecting Data

The first use of the term 'statistics' is to refer to simple numerical data. Before collecting a set of data, we must define its scope; before interpreting the data others have collected, or their research results, we need to understand the basis of their data.

In recording the daily number of occupied beds in a ward, there is no definitional problem over beds occupied by a particular in-patient for the full 24 hours of the day. But what about the days on which a patient arrives or departs and the bed is not occupied by that patient at both the beginning and the end of the day? A bed must not be counted as occupied twice on the same day, one patient occupying it in the morning before discharge, and another admitted to the same bed later in the day. What about beds for day patients? We require rules for dealing with these and other similar problems.

Relating data to time points is important. Looking at staff in post in the National Health Service (NHS), whether by hospital authority, type of staff, age, sex, grade, specialty, or any other aspect, requires a specific point in time to which the 'count' relates.

Categories or groupings are defined so that there is somewhere appropriate for every person or unit. A category described as 'other' usefully covers a few items that do not fit into the main categories. *Department of Health* (1989) *Health and Personal Social Services Statistics for England 1989*, Table 3.19, 'Professional and technical staff: Analysis by occupation', covers approximately 79,000 staff employed at 30 September 1987. There is a category 'Other scientific and professional staff'—311 in number. These included 'psychology technicians, speech therapy helpers, part-time and assistant chaplains and other scientific and professional staff'. Combining these small groups is sensible since in total they amount to approximately 0.4% or less than 4 per thousand of all professional and technical staff. An 'other' category used in this way as a 'remainder' for small disparate groups is a convenient device, but should be used sparingly.

We might wish to group patients according to their medical or surgical condition. If a patient is receiving treatment for two different conditions, do we put the patient in both categories with the attendant risk of confusion and overstatement of the total number of patients? Are we counting patients or the incidence of conditions? A decision is required.

Suppose we are studying the number of beds available to each specialty in a hospital, and there are wards that take cases for more than one specialty with numbers for each fluctuating in line with varying needs. We could consider beds in use on a particular date or dates, but what about empty beds? How should these be allocated?

Consistent rules are required for (1) defining and limiting categories, and (2) ensuring that there is one place and one place only for a particular item.

In the research field prior definition of categories is of prime importance and requires careful thought in advance of a research study. Sufficient information must be collected, and enough detail in that information. Seeking additional data after a project has started can be expensive if not impossible to achieve, and damaging in the omission. It is easier to collect information in more detail than may eventually be required, and to collapse categories. Disaggregating data and subdividing categories may be impossible. Take age as an example. It is safer to collect information on date of birth (which does not change and for which reporting is very reliable) or age in years at a particular date. Age can then be handled as required. But age recorded by ten year age groups cannot later be provided in greater detail.

In order to collect information on the length of time different categories of nursing staff had worked in the NHS, we would have to:

1. define categories of staff making sure all possible staff were covered and that each person was eligible for inclusion in one category only:
2. define the relevant period(s) of service. Is a simple aggregate required, or information about service in different categories? What about breaks in service—do we need to know anything about these, and if so what? Training periods, part-time service—how do these fit in? What is the cut-off date (service up to . . .)?

The aim is to ensure that none who should be included are omitted, and none ineligible included.

We would also be collecting other information such as sex, date of birth/ age, nursing qualifications, other educational qualifications, and possibly when the nurse first was employed in the NHS. Precisely what was required would depend on the nature and purposes of the research study. The crucial point is the need to start by taking these essential decisions.

Any information collected requires careful definitions. We should err in collecting slightly more information than may be needed rather than run the risk of omitting something essential, accepting that eventually some data might be aggregated or even discarded. Data must be collected systematically and accurately. The information obtained must be recorded and counted correctly, with careful checks.

A last reminder; when using other people's statistical material, we have to ask of their methods the questions just discussed—what the data represents, its coverage, its reliability. Only then can we make use of it.

2.2 Published Statistics

We are all aware of the flow of information, including statistical information, about all aspects of individual and community activity. Health and NHS matters are no exception. If seeking information of this kind, make use of library sources to identify it. These would include the libraries of the Royal College of Nursing and other professional bodies, the King Edward's Hospital Fund for London, the Department of Health (DH),* academic and research institutions, professional and learned societies, and major public libraries. Computers provide access to knowledge of what material exists and where it is held. There is a network of information available through the efficiency of library searches, providing an extensive and easily available data source. Before starting on such a library search seek the advice of librarians.

It is impossible to describe the published statistical data available, short of writing a substantial text on that alone. There are a number of major publications and sources. Health and Personal Social Services Statistics for England published annually by DH is exactly as described—a series of statistical tables on staff, patients, financial matters etc. Other annual publications from DH have their share of statistics. The main ones are *The Health Services in England*; the report of the Chief Medical Officer of DH, *On the State of the Public Health*; and, jointly with the Office of Population Censuses and Surveys (OPCS), *Hospital In-patient Inquiry*. There are other occasional studies published by DH (many on mental health), and the more recently introduced (1985) *Statistical Bulletin*, all of which add to the flow of data. To these are added routine records such as the causes of death and the incidence of notifiable diseases.

Not only DH is involved; OPCS publishes separate volumes on health-related topics, including for example morbidity, cancer, communicable diseases, congenital malformations and abortion. The quarterly OPCS publication *Population Trends* includes articles on health matters, supported by statistical data, and also regular tables of vital statistics.[†]

---

*The division of the Department of Health and Social Security (DHSS) into its original constituent parts of Health and Social Security in 1988 adds some confusion to library searches. Material previously published by DHSS will be under that authorship. Currently, health information will be under the authorship of DH. In this text, references to material published by DH should be taken to include earlier material published by DHSS.

[†] The statistics published in *Population Trends* include annual and quarterly statistics on population and population change, births, marriages, divorces, deaths and abortions. The death statistics include death by broad category of cause, and infant mortality, also disaggregated as stillbirths, neonatal mortality and perinatal mortality. Recent articles have covered trends in morbidity and mortality from asthma (49, Autumn 1987), winter mortality, temperature and influenza (54, Autumn 1988) and a study of triplet and higher order births (62, Winter 1990).

A section summarising data on health is included in *Social Trends*, published annually by the Central Statistical Office (CSO). The *General Household Survey* (GHS), also published annually by CSO,* includes a section on health, although the topics included in that section vary. The inclusion in the GHS of personal characteristics of individuals and household data provides useful cross-tabulations.

The annual New Earnings Survey (NES), published by the Department of Employment (DE) provides much data on the earnings of nursing staff, and other occupational groups. Many reports and studies on health matters are produced by the Royal College of Nursing, the King Edward's Hospital Fund for London and the Office of Health Economics.

Section 1 above discussed the importance of setting definitions for any statistical data to be collected. It is good practice, well followed in official government publications, to provide adequate definitions where descriptions are not sufficient. There is no doubt what is meant by a 'registered nurse', or by 'not having any natural teeth'. But 'chronic sickness' (see GHS) requires definition. The same need for definitions and demarcation lines applies to any study which involves collecting data. We need to know the terms, categories, definitions, being used. Good studies set out this information very clearly, and it is important to understand this information before using or interpreting the findings of the study.

2.3   The Nature of Data—Levels of Measurement

Data do not originate in the form set out in statistical tables. The basic information may have come from routine records (deaths by category), administrative records (date of birth and hence age of employees), work records (new patients at out-patient clinics), or questionnaires (GHS). Data can be of different basic kinds. Most importantly, we must be able to recognise the data type or level of measurement with which we are dealing so that we can handle our data appropriately. There are three levels of data measurement with which we must concern ourselves—nominal, ordinal and interval.

For examples, nominal data would be derived from the number of patients in each (named) ward of a hospital, or the number of in-patients receiving treatment within each specialty in the hospital. Although there would be conventions for the ordering of the list of the wards (alphabetic, by location in different hospital wings etc.) and of the specialties (grouped by medical, surgical and psychiatric categories separately) this order is really immaterial. It has been chosen for convenience and ease of management,

---

*The GHS covers a broad range of information on health, with specific topics covered irregularly. Health and drinking patterns were covered in 1986, 1984 and 1982, and the prevalence of tinnitus in 1981.

but equally it could be altered. What matters is that patients have been allocated to named categories; the data is nominal.

Ordinal data is logically ordered. This would cover the assessment of the severity of a condition (mild, moderate, severe, very severe), the extent of patients' satisfaction with information and advice given (very satisfied, satisfied, neither satisfied nor dissatisfied, dissatisfied, very dissatisfied). Clearly, the patient whose condition is 'mild' is less seriously ill than the patient whose condition is 'moderate', and in turn, the 'moderately' ill patient is not as seriously ill as the patient whose condition is 'severe'. There is a clear order. But there is no implication as to how the mildly and moderately ill patients relate to each other. We cannot say that a moderately ill patient is twice (or three times) as ill as the mildly ill patient; only that one has a more serious condition that the other.

The third level is interval data, where the data is arranged on a numerical scale—the age of hospital dental staff, the number of patients on general medical practitioners' lists, the number of beds in a hospital. Here there is a clear numerical relationship between different units of data; a hospital dentist aged 30 years is half the age of a hospital dentist aged 60 years; a hospital with 900 beds is three times as large as a hospital with 300 beds.

Interval data is also referred to as parametric data, because the data is based on a parameter, a measure. Nominal and ordinal data differ from interval data in this respect. To make this distinction clear, nominal and ordinal data are often referred to as non-parametric data. This is an important distinction we shall wish to use.

2.4 Frequency Distributions—Categorical Distributions

For data corresponding to any of the three levels of measurement we have discussed in section 3 above, we can establish a summary showing the original items or people aggregated in particular groups and distributed across categories. We noted that for nominal data, the order of listing the categories is determined by convention or convenience (Table 2.1). For ordinal data the categories are in a logical order (Table 3.1); for interval data, the data is ordered strictly according to a numerical scale (Table 2.2).

In each case the data has been summarised in a form which tells us how many items or people are in a particular category, that is, the frequency with which items occur within that category. For this reason, data which shows the frequency with which items are distributed across a set of categories is commonly known as a frequency distribution.

There are two broad types of frequency distribution, categorical distributions and numerical distributions. In categorical distributions, the nominal or ordinal data is defined by descriptive characteristics. These can be based on the attributes of individuals, or of groups—sex of patients, patients by severity of illness, specialty of wards. In numerical distributions, data is interval data and the groups have numerical values attached—the age of medical staff, the number of patients on general medical practitioners lists or size of hospital by number of beds. Anything that can take on numerical values is termed a variable. Here the variables are age in years, numbers of patients and number of beds.

In categorical distributions, categories must be separate and distinct and provide one place only for each item. Given a good understanding of the origins and nature of the information being collected and the purposes for which it is to be used, this should present no problems. An 'other' category will deal with small numbers of different items (see section 1 above). If this contains more than 5% of total items, consider setting up additional specific categories, or adjusting existing categories to include some of the 'other' items. Table 2.1 covers all hospital nursing staff.

Table 2.1 Hospital nursing staff, England: analysis by grade

30 September   whole-time equivalents

	1982	1983	1984	1985	1986	1987
Qualified						
Senior nurses 1–5 ⎤	6,267	⎰ 221	268	264	440	654
Senior nurses 6–8 ⎦		⎱5,411	5,611	5,744	5,458	5,428
Tutorial nursing staff	3,768	4,307	4,701	4,570	4,935	5,030
Other reg. nurses	94,454	95,955	97,648	101,235	104,613	107,187
Enrolled nurses	64,044	65,401	66,466	67,460	66,875	66,074
All qualified nurses	168,534	171,295	174,693	179,273	182,319	184,373
Learners						
Post-registration	1,991	1,959	1,959	1,983	2,169	1,950
Post-enrolment	2,093	1,674	1,475	1,572	1,648	1,521
Pre-registration	50,673	50,535	50,963	49,422	48,350	47,370
Pupil nurses	20,552	18,336	15,094	12,333	10,358	8,310
All learners	75,309	72,505	69,492	65,310	62,524	59,151
Unqualified						
Other nursing staff	88,107	86,097	84,053	85,357	85,981	87,644
Cadets	161	69	30	18	6	5
All unqualified staff	88,268	86,165	84,083	85,375	85,987	87,649
All hospital nursing staff	332,111	329,965	328,268	329,959	330,830	331,172

Source: DH (1989) *Health and Personal Social Services Statistics for England 1989*, HMSO.
Note: The totals may not equal exactly the sum of subgroups, due to rounding of whole-time equivalents.

Note the following points:

1. the scope is England;
2. the units are whole-time equivalents to accommodate part-time staff. This allows comparison between groups and over time;
3. there are three major categories of hospital nursing staff—qualified, learners and unqualified, which are themselves further subdivided. Within each category the subdivisions are distinct and without overlap;

4. note that post-registration student nurses (learners) are also registered nurses, so they could 'qualify' for both categories (similarly for post-enrolment student nurse learners who are also enrolled nurses). These nurses are classified according to their current situation in the NHS as learners rather than registered or enrolled nurses;
5. categories might be amalgamated. Nursing cadets could be amalgamated with unqualified nurses since they are few in number and declining.

There are examples of categorical distributions to be found in *Health and Personal Social Services Statistics for England* and in *Social Trends*, as well as in many other publications. The categories may be given in absolute numbers or in percentages, or in both. The aim is to convey information about patterns, differences and change.

2.5 Frequency Distributions—Numerical Distributions

We have referred to interval data derived from the numerical variables of age, number of patients on general medical practitioners lists, size of hospital by number of beds. The use of frequency distributions requires ways of describing their characteristics.

The groups of a frequency distribution are called 'classes'. Sometimes a 'group' consists of a single value; more often the group covers a range of values. Table 2.2 has been adapted from *Health and Personal Social Services Statistics for England 1989*, and for the four Thames RHAs shows the number and percentage of principals in general medical practitioner partnerships of different size, and the list size of individual principals. The practice size is 1 principal, 2 principals etc. to 5 or more principals.* So for 1, 2, 3 and 4 principals there are single value classes. Since the class '5 or more principals' has no upper value, it is an open-ended class, a convenient way of accommodating values which are scattered, perhaps including a few extreme values. The open-ended class is like the 'other' class of a categorical distribution.

Turning to the list sizes in numbers of patients, the ranges of values are under 1,000 patients, 1,000 to 1,499 patients, 1,500 to 1,999 patients, continuing by steps of 500 patients until the last class—3,000 patients and over. Looking at the class 1,000 to 1,499 patients as an example, the two extreme values, 1,000 and 1,499 are called 'class limits' because they represent the lower and upper limits of the values contained in that class.

---

* Note the high proportion of principals in practices which consist of 5 or more principals—for England as a whole 35%, with the lowest figure for any individual RHA being 23%. There is an argument here for adding further size categories, say 5 and 6 principals separately, leaving '7 or more' as a final category. If this were done, the changes taking place in the size of partnerships would be clearer.

Table 2.2   General medical practitioners: Thames RHAs

1 October 1987   number/percentage of principals

		N West	N East	S East	S West
Number of principals in partnerships					
with 1 principal	number	339	386	297	153
	percentage	(17)	(19)	(15)	(10)
with 2 principals	number	334	392	366	254
	percentage	(17)	(20)	(19)	(17)
with 3 principals	number	438	399	399	228
	percentage	(22)	(20)	(21)	(15)
with 4 principals	number	256	340	312	292
	percentage	(13)	(17)	(16)	(19)
with 5 or more	number	604	475	559	610
principals	percentage	(31)	(24)	(29)	(40)
All principals		1,971	1,992	1,933	1,537
Principals with list sizes					
under 1,000 patients		57	61	42	27
1,000–1,499 patients		154	159	176	67
1,500–1,999 patients		681	675	634	525
2,000–2,499 patients		770	711	719	656
2,500–2,999 patients		215	276	301	212
3,000 patients and over		94	110	61	50
All list sizes		1,971	1,992	1,933	1,537

Source: DH (1989) *Health and Personal Social Services Statistics for England 1989*, HMSO.
Note: Percentages do not always add up to 100 due to rounding.

Note the two open-ended classes and that in contrast to the class '5 or more principals' there are relatively few lists of under 1,000 patients or of 3,000 or more patients.

Frequency distributions are used in further calculations which require a specific value to 'represent' all values in a class. That is easy for the single value classes of 1, 2, 3 and 4 principals in general medical practices. What about '5 or more principals'? Some practices will certainly have more than 5 principals, but how many principals and how many practices? Lacking information, we can only make a reasonably sensible decision; perhaps 6, or 5.5, or maybe 6.5? * Without evidence that there are many large practices of 7 or more principals we should be cautious about using any higher value. More evidence would help, in particular additional single value classes so that the open-ended class contained fewer principals.[†]

---

* We are not restricted to a whole number. A reasonable approximation is required to cover all items in a class; we use whatever seems sensible.

† Further information is available in *Health and Personal Services Statistics for England 1989*, Table 3.24. Out of 8,837 principals in partnerships of 5 or more, nearly 57% were in partnerships of 6 or more principals. So for the class '5 or more principals', 6 would be a reasonable representative value.

Ignoring for the moment the open-ended classes, each class covers a particular range of values. For a representative value, the convention is to take the midpoint between the lowest and highest values included in the class (that is, the midpoint of the class limits). The class midpoint (or the single value in a class) is the value used to represent all in that class. The midpoint between 1,000 and 1,499 is 1,249.5; between 1,500 and 1,999 is 1,749.5. And so on. The numbers of principals with list sizes in the open-ended classes are relatively small. Most small lists are likely to be fairly close to 1,000 patients, with very few lists below 500 patients. We would be unwise to take a value below 749.5 (the value in sequence with the higher classes) as the representative value for this class, and any number up to 900 or even 950 could be reasonable. Similarly large lists are unlikely to be greatly in excess of 3,000 patients. Probably the value in sequence, 3,249.5 patients is the highest we should consider for a representative value; one lower by 100 or so patients could be equally acceptable. The decision on the representative value for an open-ended class is subjective, but choice must be informed and sensible.

Another measure required is the class interval, the range or size group covered by a particular class. For the data on the size of general medical practitioners' lists, and ignoring the open-ended classes, the class intervals are all 500 patients. The easiest way of getting the class interval is to look at the sequence of the lower values of the classes. Here this sequence is 1,000, 1,500, 2,000, 2,500. The increase is 500 patients each time, and the interval for all these classes is 500 patients.*

2.6 Continuous and Discrete Distributions

For interval data, there are two kinds of variables, continuous and discrete (or discontinuous). A continuous variable, for example age, takes all possible values on a continuum. I do not suddenly become exactly 34 years of age having yesterday been 33 years of age. From the 33rd anniversary of my birth my age crept by infinitely small increments to reach my 34th anniversary. On the other hand, patients and hospital beds come in whole numbers only. A general medical practitioner may one day have a list of 2,517 patients and the next day have 2,518 patients—he can never have anything in between. The same applies to hospital beds; a hospital may have 610 or 611 beds, but nothing in between. As well as age, height,

---

*Class intervals do not all have to be equal. List sizes might be 1,000 to 1,499; 1,500 to 1,749; 1,750 to 1,999; 2,000 to 2,499. The lowest values are 1,000; 1,500; 1,750; 2,000. The class interval for the first class is 500 patients but for the second and third is 250 patients, reverting to 500 for the next class. Class intervals often do vary in size but are usually in simple multiple relationship, such as 250, 500 and 1,000.

weight, temperature, time and speed are examples of continuous variables. The great majority of variables are discrete (or discontinuous); they take on specific values only. Examples are number of patients, number of staff, number of hospital beds and number of out-patient sessions.

Whether a variable is continuous or discrete, information is collected and handled as if the variable were discrete. Take the continuous variable weight. If weighing patients in hospital, it could be to the nearest half kilogram (approximately one pound). This puts the data on exactly the same basis as the number of patients on general medical practitioners' lists or the number of beds in a hospital. Patients will be recorded as weighing 72.0 kg, 72.5 kg, 73.0 kg etc. with no weights recorded in between. Their weight is being measured in the specific unit half kilogram. For discrete variables the unit of measurement usually settles itself—patients, staff, hospital beds and out-patient sessions are straightforward enough, but for continuous variables a positive decision is required about the unit of measurement. Should patients be weighed in kilograms, or half kilograms, or even quarter kilograms? It is a practical decision (babies would be weighed using a much smaller unit of measurement than for adults).

Mathematically all variables are treated as continuous. It does not fit with the mathematical handling of data to have only limited specific values. Go back to Table 2.2 and list sizes of general medical practitioners. The list sizes include 1,000 to 1,499 and 1,500 to 1,999. On the continuous scale there is a 'gap' between 1,499 and 1,500. To treat data as being on a continuous scale each class is extended to the middle of the 'gap'. So 1,000 to 1,499 becomes 999.5 to 1,499.5; and 1,500 to 1,999 becomes 1,499.5 to 1,999.5. Why bother about this? Firstly (a theoretical reason), because we need to understand how the data behave; and secondly (a practical reason), because we may need to know where a class begins and ends on the continuous scale. These points (999.5, 1,499.5, 1,999.5 etc.) are known as class boundaries; they are the points where two classes meet, and are always points where no actual values are recorded. The class boundary (e.g. 1,499.5) is the upper class boundary of the class below it (1,000 to 1,499), and the lower class boundary of the class above it (1,500 to 1,999).

The difference of 0.5 of a patient is hardly material when looking at list sizes of general medical practitioners which are measured in hundreds of patients. Where ranges of values are much smaller, the difference will be important. If length of in-patient stay is recorded using classes 1–2 days, 3–5 days, 6–10 days, the half day difference on the continuous scale would certainly matter. Here classes would be 0.5–2.5 days, 2.5–5.5 days, 5.5–10.5 days.

Values on the continuous scale also make class intervals clearer. For the number of patients, the difference between the class boundaries of 999.5 and 1,499.5 is 500—the correct class interval. Note that the class interval is *not* the difference between 1,000 and 1,499, the class limits. Commonsense would suggest that 499 is a most unlikely class interval. On the continuous scale for length of in-patient stay (1–2, 3–5 and 6–10 days), the class intervals are 2 days, 3 days and 5 days (not 1, 2 and 4 days).

The same principles apply to both discrete and continuous variables. Consider the continuous variable weight to the nearest half kilogram. The class boundaries will be midway between the class limits. So for classes of 70.0–74.5 kg, 75.0–79.5 kg, 80.0–84.5 kg etc., measuring in units of 0.5 kg, the boundaries would be at 69.75 kg, 74.75 kg, 79.75 kg, 84.75 kg and so on, clearly demonstrating a class interval of 5 kg. Knowing about class boundaries is part of being able to handle data on a continuous scale.

We need to understand about class boundaries, although they are seldom used directly. Operationally class limits are required for grouping data and for determining the midpoint; the class interval is also required for computations.

2.7   Structuring Frequency Distributions

Here are some guidelines for setting out interval data in a frequency distribution:

1. start with some approximation (usually available) of the range of values covered by the variable (e.g. age in years varying from 20 to 70, size of general medical practitioners' lists varying between 500 and 3,500 patients);
2. consider where most of the values are likely to be concentrated (see 3 below);
3. think of dividing the range of values (1 above) into suitable groupings—classes. A common class interval throughout is not essential. Narrower class intervals might be better where the data are more concentrated. All class intervals should be a simple multiple of the smallest unless there are very good reasons to the contrary;*
4. if in doubt start off with class intervals which are smaller than might eventually be needed. Classes can always be aggregated; it may be impossible to disaggregate the data if the initial classes are too big;

---

* *Health and Personal Social Services Statistics for England 1989*, Table 4.2 covers size of hospital by number of beds. The smallest class is open-ended (under 50 beds); the others are 200 (50–249 beds), 250 (250–499 beds), 500 (500–999 beds) and 1,000 (1,000–1,999 beds).

There is an interesting age grouping in Table 6.6 on District nursing services, the age of patient when first treated. The groups are under 5 years, 5–16 years, 17–64 years, 65 years and over. The group 5–16 years covers those of compulsory school age, and 65 years is the dividing line separating out 'the elderly'. There are good reasons for these particular age-groups.

5. no single class should contain a high proportion of the total items. A frequency in one class of 20% or more should be scrutinised—should the class be subdivided? There may be good reasons for leaving it as it is, but this needs checking; *

6. a small number of scattered extreme values at either or both ends of the distribution can be accommodated by using open-ended classes (as in Table 2.2 above);

7. the number of classes used depends on the type of data, the purpose of classification, and the other uses to which the distribution may be put. Too many classes can be confusing and the 'pattern' shown by the data unclear. Too few could mean loss of information, so that the data would not be so helpful. A rough guide is not less than 6 classes, not more than 12.

A critical look at the intended structure of a frequency distribution will ensure that it conveys the information we require.

2.8   Summary

● You understand the importance of clear definitions when classifying and collecting data, and of exploring the definitions used when studying published data.

● You are aware of some major sources of statistical information.

● In looking at data you understand the difference between categorical and frequency distributions, between nominal, ordinal and interval data, between continuous and discrete distributions, and what is meant by a variable.

● You are able to define and obtain (from a frequency distribution):

   1. class limits
   2. class boundaries
   3. class intervals
   4. class midpoints.

Further Reading

Study the way in which data have been handled in published documents. Published statistics referred to in section 2 above make a starting point.

---

* In Table 2.2 above, the general medical practitioner list sizes show substantial numbers in the group 2,000–2,499. Between one third and one half of all lists fall within this range. Lists of 1,500–1,999 are nearly as common. This is an expected concentration, but could there be an argument for dividing these groups into smaller classes?

Note the points listed in section 3 when looking at tables. It is common practice, always followed in official government publications, to describe methodology and set out definitions used. Read these sections, especially the definitions relating to any table you are studying.

A Little Practice

1. The heights of 420 student nurses are measured to the nearest centimetre, and the following distribution obtained:

Height in metres	Number of student nurses
1.55 to 1.59	16
1.60 to 1.64	68
1.65 to 1.69	156
1.70 to 1.74	119
1.75 to 1.79	40
1.80 to 1.84	18
1.85 to 1.89	3
All student nurses	420

(a) Is this a discrete or continuous distribution?
(b) What is the variable? And what is the unit of measurement?
(c) What are the class limits for the classes of the distribution?
(d) And the class boundaries?
(e) And the class midpoints?
(f) Is the class interval the same for all classes? What is/are the class interval(s)?

2. Over a period of 30 days, the daily number of beds occupied in two wards of 25 beds was recorded. The results were as follows:

Beds occupied	Ward A	Ward B
10 to 15	2	1
16 to 17	3	2
18 or 19	5	6
20 or 21	7	8
22 or 23	8	9
24 or 25	5	4
	30	30

Answer the same questions about this set of data as for question 1.

3. The number of out-patient visits paid by 90 out-patients to the completion of treatment was recorded for a particular clinic, with the following results:

Number of out-patient visits	Number of patients
one	5
two	14
three	28
four	24
five	11
six, seven or eight	8
All out-patients	90

Answer the same questions for this set of data as for question 1.

3

Graphs and Other Visual Aids

3.1 Line Graphs

Grouping and tabulating data is not the only way of conveying information. Visual presentation offers a broad rather than a detailed picture. A commonly used form is line graphs. Graphs show major changes, whether values are rising or falling, whether change is steady, accelerating or declining. They are particularly useful for showing changes over time (commonly known as a time series), and are suitable also for ordinal and interval data.

A graph may consist of a single line (usually a time series), or several graph lines, for purposes of comparison. Multiple graphs can show different absolute levels of a variable, and whether numbers in some groups are rising or falling more or less rapidly than others. Where several graph lines are shown on the same diagram, they should be sufficiently clear to permit proper comparisons and interpretations. Confused, crossing and re-crossing graph lines are not helpful and another form of presentation should be chosen, for example, bar charts (see section 3.2).

Taking data from Table 2.1 on hospital nursing staff, a graph showing the sub-total for the three major categories will emphasise what is happening to the composition of nursing staff. Figure 3.1 shows graph lines for total hospital nursing staff, and for qualified, learners and unqualified staff separately.

Whilst the total number of hospital nursing staff has varied little between 1982 and 1987, the relative importance of the different subgroups has changed considerably. Qualified nurses (more than half the total of all hospital nursing staff) have increased in number steadily over this period, but their increase has been matched by a corresponding decline in learners. There has been some variation in unqualified nursing staff, but their numbers have remained relatively constant.

A different and more complex approach to graphs is possible.

Table 3.1 covers persons aged 18 years and over; the data is derived from the GHS, and the drinking habits are defined in the Appendix to *Social Trends*.

The graph lines in Figure 3.2a and b are cumulative; the graph lines for moderate drinkers cover also heavier drinkers, the lines for frequent

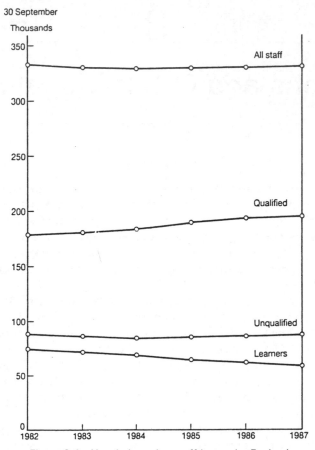

30 September

Thousands

Figure 3.1   Hospital nursing staff by grade, England

drinkers include both moderate and heavier drinkers. The vertical gap
between the lines for moderate and heavier drinkers represents the percentage of moderate drinkers. A dividing line can be set at any level, whether for
example between those who are abstainers or occasional drinkers, and all
others, or say between moderate or heavier drinkers, and all others. This is
a suitable graph where the categories are on an ordinary scale. In this
example the changes in drinking habits and the differences between men
and women are shown much more clearly by the graphs than by the data
itself. Compared with women, a higher percentage of men are moderate
or heavier drinkers. But the underlying trend is for a modest decline in
drinking by males. For women, the picture is different, suggesting very
little, if any, change in the drinking patterns of women. Indeed there is a
hint of a slight increase in drinking by women, but the changes are very
small and could easily be accounted for by sampling error (see Chapter 12).

Table 3.1 Drinking habits by sex, Great Britain

Percentages

Type of drinker	Males				Females			
	1978	1980	1982	1984	1978	1980	1982	1984
Abstainer	5	5	6	7	11	12	12	13
Occasional	9	9	10	9	25	22	23	20
Infrequent light	11	12	12	12	19	19	20	19
Frequent light	34	37	37	38	39	41	40	42
Moderate	15	14	14	14	4	4	4	4
Heavier	25	23	21	20	2	2	1	2
Sample size (numbers)	10,015	9,959	8,870	8,070	11,650	11,557	10,185	9,430

Source: CSO (1988) *Social Trends 18 1988* HMSO.

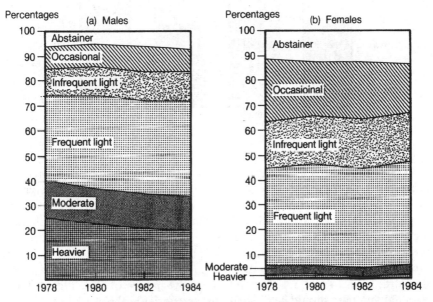

Figure 3.2 Drinking habits by sex, Great Britain

3.2 Bar Charts

Bar charts are an alternative to graphs. These can take several forms, in that comparison can be within a single bar, and also between bars. The diagrams illustrating this section are of bars broken down into categories or components, and which may be referred to as component bar charts. Consider the data from Table 2.2. The numbers of principals in partnerships of different size are shown in Figure 3.3.

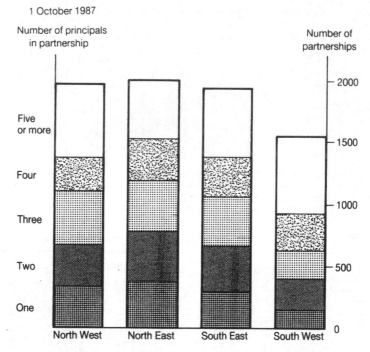

Figure 3.3 General medical practitioners: Thames RHAs

In diagrams, area is always pro-rata to the absolute numbers or to percentages. In these bars, the base size is common to all and the height of the rectangle is proportionate to the total number of principals in the RHA. The bars themselves are divided into categories or components with each segment proportionate to the number of principals in the partnership size. If showing percentages, each rectangle is the same height with the height of the segments proportionate to the percentage of principals in each partnership size, as in Figure 3.4. Depending on the nature of the data, it is not essential that bars should be divided into categories in this way, but showing the size of different component categories is part of illustration and comparison.

The emphasis in Figure 3.3 is on the differences between the four Thames RHAs in terms of the numbers of principals in each partnership size. The total number of principals is quite close as between the NW, NE and SE Thames RHAs, but in the SW Thames RHA, there are many fewer. Figure 3.4 brings out another point; that the pattern of partnerships in the SW Thames RHA is broadly different from that in the other three. In the SW Thames RHA, the majority of principals are in partnerships of four or more; in the other three, the majority are in partnerships of three or less. The differences are quite marked and well demonstrated in Figure 3.4.

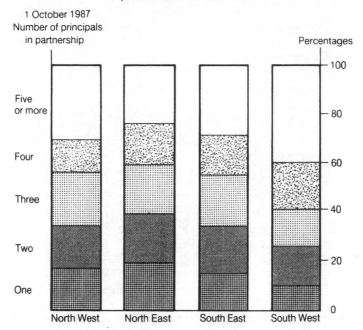

Figure 3.4   General medical practitioners: Thames RHAs

A single bar is best divided into a few categories only; as a rough guide, six categories is a reasonable maximum number into which to divide a single bar.

The data on Hospital nursing staff from Table 2.1 could not helpfully be presented as single bars for each year. There are initially ten separate categories. If the smallest were amalgamated (creating all senior nurses, all post-registration/enrolment learners, all unqualified nursing staff), there would remain seven categories. Even so, in a single bar for each year, the differences and changes would hardly show up because of the small scale involved. A more complex way of presenting this data is Figure 3.5.

Information is grouped over the six years, firstly for qualified nurses, secondly for learners and thirdly for unqualified nursing staff. As this is based on numbers of staff, the heights of the bars indicate what is happening to the total number of staff in each category. The bar charts show the *general* pattern of change in these three groups over the six years—qualified nurses rising, learners declining and unqualified staff approximately constant. In more detail we note that the growth in qualified nurses is only marginally in senior nurses, mainly in other registered nurses. Amongst learners there is an overall decline, most marked in pupil nurses, but also in pre-registration nurses. Post-registration and post-enrolment learners are very small and almost constant in number.

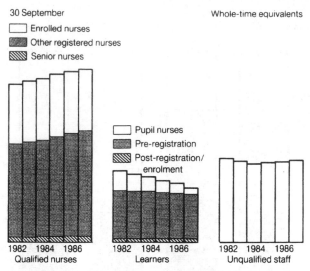

Figure 3.5   Hospital nursing staff by grade, England

The grouped arrangement of the bar charts provides some useful comparative information. Whereas Table 2.1 emphasises that the total of all hospital nursing staff has changed little over these six years, the bar charts illustrate changes in the underlying pattern.

Compare Figure 3.5 with the line graphs in Figure 3.1. Which do you think is the more useful for this information?

3.3   Pie Charts

This is a good moment to consider pie charts. A pie chart is a circle divided into 'slices' or 'segments' which are proportionate either to numbers or to percentages in different categories. Pie charts are used comparatively in much the same way as bar charts. It is more common to have the segments based on percentages than on absolute numbers. The circles are then the same size, and divided into segments pro rata to the percentage distribution. Comparison between the segments in equal sized pie charts is easy. The alternative is to vary the size of the circle so that each is proportionate to the absolute number it represents. Unfortunately this raises the problem of comparing segments of pies (circles) of different sizes. Which is bigger, a large slice of a small pie or a small slice of a large pie? As a rule of thumb, use pie charts only for percentage distributions. The pie charts in Figure 3.6 are based on the data for learners for 1983, 1985 and 1987.

The distributional changes show clearly. As a *proportion* of total learners, post-registration and post-enrolment learners are increasing marginally, pre-registration learners are increasing substantially and pupil

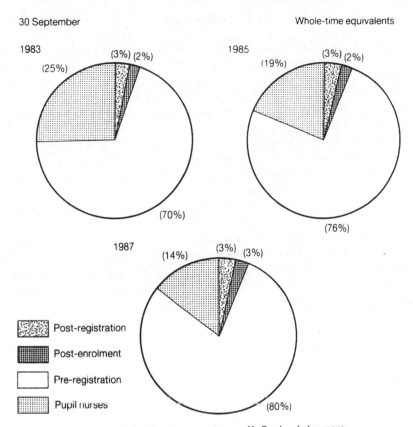

30 September   Whole-time equivalents

Figure 3.6 Hospital nursing staff, England: learners

nurses declining rapidly (as would be expected with current training policy changes). What we must not ignore is what is happening to *absolute* numbers of learners (Table 2.1 and Figure 3.5). Here there is a different story; total learners are *declining* in number and most importantly this is happening to pre-registration learners as well as to pupil nurses. This illustrates the need to look at data both as percentage distributions and as absolute numbers.

The potential advantage of pie charts over bar charts is that the smaller categories, and the changes in them, show more clearly. The catch is that pie charts are a little tedious to construct.*

---

* In constructing a pie chart, you need a protractor to measure the angle (size of each sector) from the centre of the circle. To get the number of degrees for a particular sector, multiply the percentage for each subgroup (to one place of decimals) by 3.6. Round to the nearest whole number, and that is the size of the sector in degrees. With a pair of compasses, draw circles of equal size for each data set. Keep the order of the sectors the same, using a common starting point in each circle. If you wish to have circles proportionate to the absolute totals involved, then the radius of each circle must be proportionate to the *square root* of the respective totals. Perhaps bar charts would be easier!

3.4   Histograms

Histograms are the block diagrams used for frequency distributions (interval data), with variable values along the horizontal axis, and frequencies along the vertical axis. The blocks are correctly scaled, the base of each being proportionate to the class interval, the range of values covered. Figure 3.7 is based on the list sizes for general medical practitioners in the NW Thames RHA from Table 2.2.

Area represents frequency. All groups are the same size (class interval 500 patients),* therefore each rectangle has the same base length, and the height of the rectangle is proportionate to the number of general medical practitioners with list sizes within each range.

As another example, we can construct a histogram for the size of general medical practices. In Table 2.2 we noted the problem of the open-ended class '5 or more principals'. If this is taken as '5 or 6 principals', the height of the rectangle on a double-sized base would be proportionate to *half* the number of principals (604/2 = 302), so that the area of the rectangle is still proportionate to the frequency of 604. Alternatively, since a high proportion (31%) of principals are in practices of 5 or more principals, we

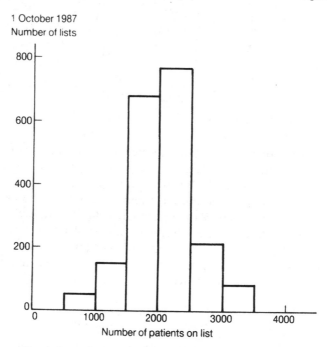

Figure 3.7   General medical practitioners NW Thames RHA

---

* The open-ended classes have been taken as 500–999 and 3,000–3,499 patients.

might consider it more realistic to take the practice size as '5, 6 or 7' principals. This would require a base three times the size of the base for the other single value classes. We would have to divide the frequency for '5 or more principals' by 3 to get the height of the rectangle (604/3 = 201.3). Both these alternatives are shown in Figure 3.8a and b. The second alternative, Figure 3.8b, may be a more realistic presentation of the data.

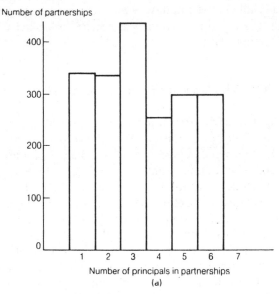

(a)

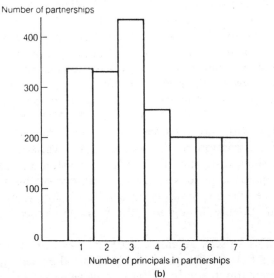

(b)

Figure 3.8 Principals by size of general medical practice: NW Thames RHA 1987

A histogram demonstrates the distribution of numerical frequency data; it is the pattern *within* the data which is of interest. Comparison between histograms is possible, but not by superimposing one upon the other which can only be confusing.

A final point: Graphs and diagrams are aids in presenting information. If they are helpful, then we use them. Many readers are helped by visual presentation, especially in the emphasis which this can give to major aspects of the data. But graphs and diagrams are not to be looked upon as substitutes for the original data.

3.5   The Choice of Visual Presentation

The nature of the data and information to be conveyed largely determines the final choice of visual presentation. We take into account whether the data are in numbers or percentages, whether simple or complex (more than two variables), and what comparisons are required.

Graphs are particularly useful for time series where the data are in absolute numbers (Figure 3.1) or cumulative percentages (Figure 3.2). They are a simple and easily understood form of visual presentation.

In their various forms, bar charts are the most flexible method of presentation, since they can take into account several variables. Bar charts can be used for time series data, especially where more elaborate comparison is desired between groups for each time point, and an additional variable or variables are involved (Figure 3.5). The data here are more complex than could be handled through a graph.

Pie charts are fine for showing percentage frequency distributions, and can be used either to show a single distribution, or comparatively for two or more distributions (Figure 3.6). They have a positive advantage for categorical data, or where the size of any one or more category is small. They are inappropriate for comparisons based on absolute numbers, or for complex data.

Histograms deal with interval data. Their aim is to show the pattern *within* the data, in relation to the values of the variable. Histograms normally cover a single distribution, although two histograms can be shown together for comparative purposes. Overlapping two histograms to make comparison between them is basically unsuccessful as the visual impression is very confused. So use histograms for a single numerical frequency distribution.

Finally, remember to seek guidance from the way in which experienced statisticians have selected and used methods of visual presentation, accompanied by comment on the information conveyed thereby (see Further Reading below).

3.6 Summary

- You have now covered the main diagrammatic forms for showing data.
- You are able to construct and interpret:

1. line graphs
2. bar charts
3. pie charts
4. histograms

Further Reading

CSO *Social Trends*, HMSO has already been referred to as a useful source of guidance; look at the most recent issue, in particular the section on Health and Personal Social Services. Look at the relationship between the statistical tables, graphs etc. and discussion in the text.

Other CSO publications with health sections which use visual presentation are *Population Trends* and the *General Household Survey*.

Serious journals (including the nursing and medical press) and newspapers frequently illustrate articles with graphs or bar charts, so note the uses here.

For an additional view: Hannagan T J (1988 2nd edn) *Mastering Statistics* Chapters 7 and 8. Basingstoke: Macmillan.

A Little Practice

Use A4 millimetre graph paper for these examples.

1. The daily number of occupied beds over a two week period in two 40-bed wards was recorded.

Day	Ward A	Ward B	Day	Ward A	Ward B
1	37	32	8	35	32
2	36	34	9	38	33
3	34	36	10	38	35
4	34	36	11	37	38
5	32	38	12	39	39
6	35	37	13	38	36
7	34	35	14	39	36

Draw graph lines for the number of occupied beds in each ward on the same sheet of graph paper. Be careful, the lines cross over, and different coloured lines would help to make this clear. Use 1 cm to represent one day on the horizontal axis, and to represent two beds on the vertical axis. Remember to give a title to your graph, to name the variable and the units, and to label the graph lines.

2. The age in years of 35 patients on Day 6 in Ward A is as follows:

Under 30 years	3
30 and under 45 years	8
45 and under 60 years	15
60 years and over	9

Draw a simple bar chart to illustrate this information. Use 4 cm for the base of your bar, and 5 mm on the vertical scale to represent 1 patient.

3. Display the data from question 1, Chapter 2 (the height of student nurses) as a histogram. Use 2 cm on the horizontal scale to equal 5 cm height (0.05 ms), and use 1 cm on the vertical scale to equal 10 student nurses.

4

The Interpretation of Tables

4.1 Simple Arithmetic Aids—Percentages, Ratios

Chapters 2 and 3 covered the organisation of data in frequency distributions and the role of visual aids. The next step is to be able to look at tables containing data, and to appreciate quickly and easily the information contained therein. There are two broad aspects to consider; firstly, what the table shows as it stands; and secondly, since comparisons between figures can be difficult using only original absolute numbers, what further information is conveyed by simple calculations, such as percentages or ratios. Table 4.1a (taken from DH (1989) *Health and Personal Social Services Statistics for England 1989*, HMSO) illustrates these points.

The table shows the total number of general dental practitioners divided by sex for the years 1983 to 1988 inclusive. Clearly, (1) the total number of general dental practitioners has gone up each year compared with the previous year, and (2) this is true for each sex separately. But what is happening to the relative numbers of male and female general dental practitioners? Ways of exploring this are shown in Table 4.1b, c and d.

Table 4.1 General dental practitioners by sex, England

30 September

	1983	1984	1985	1986	1987	1988
a Number of practitioners						
Male	11,604	11,828	11,916	11,946	11,984	12,062
Female	2,068	2,238	2,418	2,570	2,781	3,008
Total	13,672	14,066	14,334	14,516	14,765	15,070
b Percentages						
Male	84.9	84.1	83.1	82.3	81.2	80.0
Female	15.1	15.9	16.9	17.7	18.8	20.0
Total	100.0	100.0	100.0	100.0	100.0	100.0
c Ratio male : female	5.6	5.3	4.9	4.6	4.3	4.0
d Fraction female/total	1/7	1/6	1/6	1/6	1/5	1/5

First we calculate the percentages of total general dental practitioners who are male and female respectively.

A percentage is the number of hundredth parts represented by a subgroup in relation to a total. We divide one subgroup (say male general dental practitioners for 1983) by the total of all general dental practitioners for that year and multiply by 100. This gives the number of hundredth parts:

$$\frac{11,604}{13,672} \times 100 = 84.9\%$$

This is repeated for female general dental practitioners for 1983, and for both sexes for all the other years. The results are shown in Table 4.1b.

A second approach is to calculate the ratio between males and females, giving the number of males for each female general dental practitioner. For 1983 this would be:

$$\frac{\text{males}}{\text{females}} = \frac{11,604}{2,068} = 5.6$$

For all years, the male : female ratios are shown in Table 4.1c.*

Finally we could look at female general dental practitioners (the smaller group in every year) as a fraction of the total number of general dental practitioners. This is less helpful because a fraction is more approximate than either a percentage or a ratio, but it does express a general overall relationship. For 1983 the fraction is:

$$\frac{\text{female general dental practitioners}}{\text{total general dental practitioners}} = \frac{2,068}{13,672}$$

This can be rewritten as

$$\frac{1}{13,672/2,068} = \frac{1}{6.6}$$

or approximately one seventh. The fractions for all years are shown in Table 4.1d.

The following statements are based on these measures:

1. the percentage of general dental practitioners who are female has increased each year compared with the previous year, from 15.1% in 1983 to 20.0% by 1988;

---

*In showing a relationship between male and female numbers, and examining the changes that are taking place, we can legitimately refer to males as an inexact number. Whole numbers would be too approximate.

2. the ratio of male to female general dental practitioners has declined each
   year compared with the previous year, from 5.6 in 1983 to 4.0 by 1988;
3. the fraction of general dental practitioners who were female was
   approximately one seventh of all general dental practitioners in 1983, but
   has increased to one fifth by 1988;
4. this should be seen against a year on year increase in the total of general
   dental practitioners.

The first three points make much the same comment, but in different
ways. Whilst percentages are the commonly used measures for comparisons
between groups, the ratio and the fraction can be very helpful in emphasising differences, especially where there is considerable discrepancy
between the sizes of groups.

Now go to the end of this chapter, and try some examples yourself.

4.2   The Approach to Interpretation

Tables may be dealing with a single idea or situation, but broken down by
different variables, e.g. Table 4.2 on trends in total tooth loss. Interestingly,
this table covers age as interval data, with time being ordinal and sex
nominal. Other tables cover a number of related but separate sections as
Table 4.4, a summary of NHS hospital activity. Here different types of
information have been put together to provide a multidimensional picture,
each item contributing to a rounded summary. The dividing line between
the two broad types is inevitably blurred, and some tables are more than
a single variable, with some breakdown by contributory variables or
characteristics.

Looking at tables, or indeed any statistical information, we need to know
about sources, definitions, methods of data collection and reliability.
In official published statistics, sources are clearly given. In data derived
from limited sources (e.g. *Health and Personal Social Services Statistics for
England*) main sources are usually covered in a general introduction, with
additional sources given, where applicable, for individual tables. Where
various sources are used throughout (e.g. *Social Trends*), each individual
table has its specific sources. Survey reports (as the GHS or the NES)
commonly include sections on scope and methodology, with comments on
reliability and error. Explanatory notes and definitions are provided, and
usually a copy of any questionnaire used. This applies equally to statistical
material from non-official sources. In research publications generally,
we would look for adequate description of the methodology used and a
critique of the reliability and limitations of statistical and other findings.
To understand and possibly to use published statistical material, requires a
sufficient understanding of the basis of the data and what is covered by it.

We can now consider how to approach an individual table. We must be aware of the overall nature of the data, what it encompasses, and note the following:

1. the sources of the data;
2. the coverage of the data;
3. the variables contained in the tables;
4. the units of measurement used;
5. the time point(s) to which the data relates;
6. the necessary definitions and explanations attached to the data;
7. any discontinuities, or other changes, possibly external to the data itself, but which affect the data.

Armed with this guide, we can now look at tables.

4.3　A Single Variable Table

Table 4.2 shows the percentage of adults with no natural teeth by age and sex for the years 1968, 1978, 1983, 1985 and 1987.

Table 4.2　Trends in total tooth loss, England and Wales.
Percentage of adults with no natural teeth by age and sex

Persons aged 16 and over

Age	Men					Women				
	1968*	1978*	1983	1985	1987	1968*	1978*	1983	1985	1987
16–24	1	0	0	0	0	1	0	1	0	0
25–34	6	3	1	1	1	8	4	2	2	2
35–44	16	9	6	5	3	28	14	9	6	5
45–54	36	24	18	15	12	44	33	25	19	19
55–64	61	41	36	34	32	66	56	45	44	37
65–74	78	72	59	58	52	80	76	68	63	59
75 or over	88	86	75	77	73	88	87	84	81	79
All aged 16 or over	33	24	20	19	17	40	32	29	26	24
Base = 100%										
16–24	183	316	1487	1456	1567	212	319	1496	1479	1576
25–34	253	330	1488	1559	1636	262	425	1653	1638	1764
35–44	282	346	1533	1597	1602	268	344	1526	1595	1640
45–54	208	314	1208	1187	1317	267	323	1275	1195	1319
55–64	252	312	1297	1226	1231	242	313	1419	1366	1306
65–74	147	219	962	883	968	196	274	1282	1120	1220
75 or over	57	74	471	477	518	103	161	856	885	934
All aged 16 or over	1382	1912	8446	8385	8839	1550	2163	9507	9278	9759

* Adult Dental Health Survey (Vol. 1, England and Wales 1968–1978, Table 4.3).
Source: OPCS (1989) *General Household Survey 1987*, HMSO.

This is a straightforward table. Note that as well as giving the percentages of adults with no natural teeth, the base numbers are given, the number of persons covered by the survey in each subgroup. This is very useful, because the reliability of sample percentages is dependent on the sample size (or for separate age-groups, on sub-sample size)—see discussions in Chapters 8 and subsequent chapters. The samples and sub-samples for 1968 and 1978 are much smaller than for 1983, 1985 and 1987, which could affect the implications of changes from the earlier years. Where data are based on samples we cannot conclude that real changes are occurring if percentage changes are small, unless there is an observed pattern of change as here.

Examining Table 4.2 against the points listed in section 1 above:

1. the data refer to total tooth loss—the percentages of adults with no natural teeth;
2. sources are the Adult Dental Health Survey 1968–1978 and the GHS for 1983, 1985 and 1987;
3. coverage is men and women aged 16 years and over in England and Wales;
4. the variables are sex, age in years and time;
5. the units of measurement are percentages, together with sample base— the number of persons in each subgroup covered by the survey;
6. GHS data is collected over the four quarters of each calendar year, so over the year as a whole. The time point is the middle of the year. We are not given sufficient information to deduce the time point for the two years from the Adult Dental Health Survey, 1968 and 1978, but probably a mid-year time point applies also for this data. The time span covered is long and there are clear trends which could not be upset by marginal time point differences. For an exact time point, check with the Adult Dental Health Survey;
7. definitions here raise no problems. GHS respondents were asked ". . . have you still got some of your natural teeth, or have you lost them all?" Sex and age (from date of birth) are as reported at the time of the survey.

What now? We can look at the variables individually, at how the variables run together, and whether there are associations. We can look for notable or maverick figures. We can seek to identify trends, to reach broadly applicable conclusions, to point up differences and change emphasised by the figures.

Turning again to Table 4.2. The main points that emerge are:

8. unsurprisingly, total tooth loss increases with age;
9. the percentage of all aged 16 years and over with no natural teeth has declined through each of the given years between 1968 and 1987. This is true for both sexes;

10. the percentage of each age-group with no natural teeth has also declined through each of the given years from 1968 to 1987, and this holds for both sexes; *

11. comparing all men aged 16 years and over with all women, higher percentages of women than men had no natural teeth for each of the given years;

12. this is not a function of different numbers of men and women in each age-group,[†] since with very limited exceptions (those aged 16–24 years with minimal percentages having no natural teeth, and for those aged 75 and over in 1968), there is a consistent pattern of the percentage of women having no natural teeth exceeding that for men, for all age-groups and all years;

13. the decline between 1983 and 1985 in the percentages of men with no natural teeth is very modest overall, whereas the decline for women is more marked, particularly in age-group 45–54 years (a decline from 25% to 19%) and 65–74 years (a decline from 68% to 63%);

14. but the position is different as between 1985 and 1987, when for both sexes the overall decline in the percentage with no natural teeth is 2%. The decline for men is most marked in the 65–74 years age-group (58% to 52%), and for women in the same age-group (77% to 73%) and in the 55–64 age-group (63% to 59%);

15. the data are derived from samples, so that some differences may be due to the sampling process (see Chapters 10 to 12). Between 1983 and 1985 there was a decline amongst women aged 45–54 years in the percentage with no natural teeth from 25% to 19%, but no further decline between 1985 and 1987. The apparent lack of recent improvement amongst women in this age-group may be the result of sampling error obscuring what is really a more steady decline.

16. in conclusion we would expect a future continuation of the main trend, a decline in each age-group in the percentage with no natural teeth, but that this would continue at a slower rate. The lower the starting point (percentage with no natural teeth), the more difficult it is to reduce the figure further.

Could further calculations contribute information on these two main trends? There are two possible approaches. Firstly, as between men and

---

* There is one exception to this statement, for men aged 75 years and over of whom 75% had no natural teeth in 1983, the figure for 1985 being higher at 77%. The difference is small and the percentages are derived from small samples (471 and 477 respectively). The difference between these two percentages could have arisen from the sampling process. It is not statistically significant—see Chapter 12.

† Larger numbers of elderly women than elderly men would produce a higher overall percentage of women with no natural teeth even although there were no differences between men and women by age. See Chapter 5.4 on the weighted mean.

women, we could look at the ratios of the percentages with total tooth loss, women : men, for each age-group from 35–44 years and upwards,* and for each year. This is shown in Table 4.3a.

Secondly, to examine the decline in total tooth loss for men and women separately since 1968, we could take the figures for each sex by age-group from 35–44 years as being 100 in 1968, then calculate the comparative figure for the three later years as a percentage of the 1968 figure. This is constructing an index number with 1968 = 100 as the base year. The figures for succeeding years are percentages related to the base year of 1968, and calculated as any other percentage. The excess or shortfall of each figure compared with 100 represents the percentage change since the base year of 1968. These figures are shown in Table 4.3b and c for men and women respectively.

What does this additional information contribute? All ratios in Table 4.3a are 1.00 or above indicating that the percentage of women with no

Table 4.3 Trends in total tooth loss: comparison between men and women

	1968	1978	1983	1985	1987
a Percentages with total tooth loss					
women : men					
Age in years					
35–44	1.75	1.56	1.50	1.20	1.67
45–54	1.22	1.38	1.39	1.27	1.58
55–64	1.08	1.37	1.25	1.29	1.16
65–74	1.03	1.06	1.15	1.09	1.13
75 and over	1.00	1.01	1.12	1.05	1.08
All ages	1.21	1.33	1.45	1.37	1.41
b Percentages with total tooth loss					
men (1968 = 100)					
Age in years					
35–44	100	56	38	31	19
45–54	100	67	50	42	33
55–64	100	67	59	56	52
65–74	100	92	76	74	67
75 and over	100	98	85	88	83
All ages	100	73	61	58	52
c Percentages with total tooth loss					
women (1968 = 100)					
Age in years					
35–44	100	50	32	21	18
45–54	100	75	57	43	43
55–64	100	85	68	67	56
65–74	100	95	85	79	74
75 and over	100	99	95	92	90
All ages	100	80	73	65	60

* The percentages with total tooth loss in the younger age-groups are too small to permit any meaningful comparisons.

natural teeth is equal to or above that for men in each age-group. Only women aged 35–44 years have improved their position since 1968; in other age-groups, the ratios have not declined but are higher than in 1968. Other than 55–64 years, all age-groups have higher ratios in 1987 than in 1985.

Table 4.3b and c confirm this. Again, apart from age-group 35–44 years, the decline in the percentage with no natural teeth has been sharper for men than for women, a point not clearly seen in the original table.

4.4 A Multi-variable Table

Table 4.4, which has been taken from CSO (1990) *Social Trends 20*, HMSO, provides a summary of the work of the NHS hospital service.

A multi-variable table is like a number of single variable tables put together. Following the guidance on points to be examined in section 1, and the example in section 3 above, see what information you can extract from this table. Start by listing the separate subjects covered by Table 4.4, so treating it as several single variable tables. Then examine this table in the way we looked at Table 4.2 [section 3, points (1) to (7)] to assess the basic contents of the table. Note whether your comments refer to all the data in Table 4.4, or to one of the sub-tables only. Now compare your findings with 'Table 4.4—Contents' below. Return to Table 4.4 to pick out the main items of information it contains [see section 3, points (8) to (16)]. Think about the possibilities discussed in section 2 for simple further calculations. What can you suggest? And what about a diagram or graph to emphasise a point? Think of at least one. 'Table 4.4—Information' below sets out possibilities with which to compare your ideas.

Table 4.4—Contents

1. It provides a summary of NHS hospital activities in the main areas and covers data on in-patients, including beds available and occupied; length of in-patient stay; private in-patients; day cases; and new out-patients. The data covers a number of years (1971, 1976, 1981 and 1984 to 1987);
2. the sources are various, are noted at the foot of the table, and are primarily the health departments of the four constituent countries of the UK;
3. the coverage of the table is the UK (but see footnotes);
4. the variables are patient turnover (discharges and deaths, new out-patients); work load (average, i.e. mean length of stay for in-patients; average, i.e. mean attendances per new out-patient; day case attendances; percentage of live births in hospital); resources (staffed beds available); efficiency (beds occupied, patients treated per bed available);
5. the units of measurement depend on the variable in (4) above. All units of measurement are noted against the entries in the first column. Patient

Table 4.4 National Health Service hospital summary, United Kingdom: all specialties

	1971	1976	1981	1984	1985	1986	1987[1]
All in-patients							
Discharges and deaths (thousands)	6,437	6,525	7,179	7,666	7,884	7,959	8,088
Average number of beds available daily[2] (thousands)	526	484	450	429	421	409	392
Average number of beds occupied daily (thousands)							
Maternities	19	16	15	14	13	13	13
Other patients[3]	417	378	350	333	327	316	304
Total—average number of beds occupied daily	436	394	366	347	341	330	317
Patients treated per bed available (numbers)	12.3[3]	13.6	16.0	17.8	18.7	19.4	20.6
Average length of stay (days)							
Medical patients	14.7[4]	12.1	10.2[4]	9.1	8.7	8.5	—
Surgical patients	9.1[4]	8.6	7.6[4]	6.9	6.7	6.5	—
Maternities	7.0[4]	6.7	5.6[4]	4.9	4.7	4.5	—
Percentage of live births in hospital[4]	89.8	97.6	98.9	99.0	99.1	99.1	99.2[8]
Private in-patients[5] (thousands)							
Discharges and deaths	115	95	98	79	71	—	—
Average number of beds occupied daily	2	2	1	1	1	—	—
Day case attendances (thousands)	—	565[4]	863	1,081	1,166	1,288	1,207
New out-patients[6] (thousands)							
Accidents and emergency	9,358	10,463	11,342	12,279	12,492	12,682	12,797
Other out-patients	9,572	9,170	9,816	10,376	10,604	10,758	10,350
Average attendances per new patient (numbers)[7]							
Accidents and emergency	1.6	1.6	1.4	1.4	1.3	1.3	1.3
Other out-patients	4.2	4.0	4.4	4.3	4.3	4.3	4.2

[1] 1987 figures for England relate to the financial year ending 31 March 1988.
[2] Staffed beds only.
[3] Out of the 233 thousand in-patients in England in 1987, 86 thousand were mental illness/handicap patients who occupied 40 per cent of available beds.
[4] Great Britain only.
[5] England and Wales only.
[6] The 1971 and 1976 figures for out-patients in Scotland include ancillary departments.
[7] Patients attending out-patient clinics in England solely for attention of a minor nature and not seen by a doctor, e.g. to have a dressing changed are no longer counted.
[8] United Kingdom.
Source: Department of Health, Scottish Health Service, Common Services Agency, Welsh Office, Department of Health and Social Services, Northern Ireland.

data, beds available and occupied, are given in thousands; average length of stay in days; patients treated per bed available is a number; live births in hospital are given as a percentage of all live births;

6. the data is based on aggregates or averages (means) for a calendar year;

7. definitions would be straightforward since they are related to the need to keep records of hospital activities. Note that available beds are staffed beds only. If detail is required of any of the definitions (e.g. whether in reckoning length of in-patient stay in days, the day of admission and the day of discharge were *both* counted) check at the source;

8. the footnotes note small discrepancies in the figures, which might in some circumstances be important.

Table 4.4—Information

As commented, we are looking at a whole series of separate small tables which taken together present a picture of NHS hospital activity. What changes appear over time? What points emerge?

9. The workload in terms of turnover of in-patients increased steadily between 1971 and 1987. New out-patients and day-case attendances increased between 1971 and 1986, but declined in 1987 (except for accidents and emergencies);
10. the number of patients treated per bed available increased steadily between 1971 and 1987;
11. the average number of staffed beds available daily and the average number of beds occupied daily declined between 1971 and 1987;
12. the average length of stay for all categories of in-patients declined between 1971 and 1986 (the latest figure available);
13. the percentage of live births taking place in hospital increased, reaching 99% by 1984, and still marginally rising; but note that the average number of beds occupied daily by maternity cases declined to 1985, then remained constant;
14. private in-patients have declined, both in turnover and in average number of beds occupied daily to 1986 (latest figures available);
15. new out-patients attending for accidents and emergencies rose in number, much more sharply than the rise in other new out-patients, which declined in 1987;
16. average attendances per new out-patient for accident or emergency cases have declined, but stabilised since 1985. For other new out-patients, average attendances have fluctuated, showing a very marginal decline since 1981;
17. day cases attendances, first reported in 1976, have increased very sharply, more than doubling between 1976 and 1986, and showing a slight decline in 1987.

These points all provide interesting comment on changes in NHS activity. Are useful further calculations possible here? For any of this data we might wish to look at percentage change since 1971—turning figures for later years into percentages (or indices) of the parallel figure in 1971.* This would be comparable to the calculations shown in Table 4.3b and c. Here are some examples.

1. The decline in the average length of in-patient stay for the three categories of in-patient—medical, surgical and maternities—is shown in the indices in Table 4.5a. The most rapid rate of decline has been in

---

* Any year can be taken as the base year for comparison. The base year chosen will affect the changes shown, so consider whether there is any good reason for choosing one particular year, or avoiding another.

medical cases, followed by maternities. The rate of decline has tailed off, and the scope for further decline is likely to be limited;

2. the occupancy rate for staffed beds can be studied by calculating the average (mean) daily percentage of staffed beds occupied as in Table 4.5b. It demonstrates a remarkably constant percentage rate from 1976 to 1986, varying only between 80% and 81% in all these years. The reduction in available beds has not been met by an increase in the percentage of beds occupied;

3. growth in new out-patients, especially accident and emergency cases, suggests a growth in total 'out-patient load'. But for accidents and emergencies, there has been a decline in the average attendance per new out-patient. It would be interesting to look at total out-patient attendances (new out-patients × average attendances) both for these accident and emergency cases and for other cases. These are set out in Table 4.5c and show much variation. Although all figures after 1976 are higher than the earliest year, 1971, it is unclear whether since 1976 there has really been any marked trend, upward or downward. Other out-patient attendances show a modest upward trend to 1986 but a decline in 1987, with a similar but more marked pattern in total out-patient attendances. These are also shown in Table 4.5c. A graph helps to emphasise the point (Figure 4.1).

Table 4.5 National Health Service hospital summary

	1971	1976	1981	1984	1985	1986	1987
All in-patients							
a Length of stay (days) (1971 = 100)							
Medical patients	100	82	69	62	59	58	na
Surgical patients	100	95	84	76	74	71	na
Maternities	100	96	80	70	67	64	na
b Percentage of staffed beds occupied	83	81	81	81	81	80	81
c Out-patient attendances (millions)							
Accident and emergency	15.0	16.7	15.9	17.2	16.2	16.5	16.6
Other	40.2	36.7	43.2	44.6	45.6	46.0	43.5
Total	55.2	53.4	59.1	61.8	61.8	62.5	60.1

Note: Figures not available denoted by na.

There are other possibilities we could pursue. We could turn the in-patient figure for deaths and discharges, and those for daily number of available beds into index numbers (1971 = 100). This would show very clearly the rate of increase in the turnover of patients compared with the decline in available beds. These index numbers could also be shown as graphs.

The set of data does not lend itself to presentation in bar charts or pie charts because most is simple summary information; any could be shown as graphs over time.

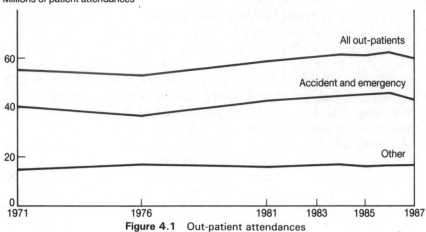

Millions of patient attendances

Figure 4.1   Out-patient attendances

These suggestions are not meant to be exhaustive of the possible ways of extending examination of Table 4.4, but examples of what we can do. The more we know about the basic data, and what they are about, the more successful we shall be in extracting useful information from tables.

4.5   Summary

- You are able to look at a table, and to extract information from it in a methodical way.
- You have learnt to carry out simple calculations of percentages, ratios etc.
- You have extended your examination of tables by using these simple measures to enhance the information obtainable.
- You can use figures from tables to produce graphs or bar charts or other visual forms which emphasise points in the data.

Further Reading

The tables in CSO *Social Trends* (HMSO) are accompanied by text which directs attention to the main point(s) of tables. Look at these, and also at articles in recent issues. (Try subjecting tables to the exercise of section 4 above before reading the text.)

More specialised are the articles in CSO *Population Trends* (HMSO); these also provide examples of tables presenting findings with discussion of the data.

Jowell R *et al.* (eds) (1990) *British Social Attitudes the 7th Report* (Aldershot: Gower), describes various aspects of British society and provides tables giving the research results with comment and discussion of the findings. The 7th report contains a chapter 'Recipes for health' about attitudes to food and eating habits.

A Little Practice

1. Using the table on the heights of student nurses (Chapter 2, question 1), calculate the percentages for the number of each height (a) to one decimal place, and (b) to whole numbers.

2. Convert the daily number of beds occupied in Ward A (Chapter 2, question 2) into percentages. Decide whether to calculate them to whole numbers or one decimal place. Why did you take this decision? (Note that percentages do not always add to 100 due to rounding.)

3. Out-patient attendances at a clinic are recorded for new patients and returning patients:

Clinic session	New patients	Returning patients
1	8	23
2	12	31
3	11	27
4	10	32
5	7	25
6	9	28
7	10	26
8	13	27
9	11	25
10	9	22

Calculate (to two decimal places) the ratio of old patients to new patients for each clinic session. This gives you the number of old patients attending for every one new patient.

4. The following data set out the available beds in ten wards in a hospital, and the mean bed-occupancy over a calendar year:

Ward	Available beds	Mean bed-occupancy
1	12	10.4
2	12	9.9
3	15	12.5
4	15	13.3
5	18	15.4
6	20	16.0
7	20	18.1
8	20	17.6
9	25	23.2
10	25	21.8

Treating the available beds as a base of 100, calculate the index (as a whole number) for the mean bed-occupancy for each ward. (Obtain the ratio of mean bed-occupancy/available beds multiplied by 100.)

Part II

Descriptive Statistics

5

Central Measures:
Measures of Location —
Mean, Median and Quantiles

5.1 The Role of Central Measures

Chapters 2 to 4 were concerned with original data and summarised data. To this information can be added the central measure which is a single value 'representative' of the data and in some way 'centrally' placed, with data values above and below it. Central measures are called 'averages'; the common 'average' is the arithmetic mean. Unless there is good reason to the contrary, assume that an average is the arithmetic mean.

Central measures enable two or more sets of data to be compared; for a single data set, comparisons can be made over time. A series of daily bed-occupancy figures for a ward does not permit easy comparison with similar figures for another ward, or for the same ward at different dates. Weekly or monthly averages (means) will show much more clearly whether changes are taking place: whether the bed-occupancy rate is higher or lower in Ward A compared with Ward B. For Ward A alone, the average bed-occupancy for successive weeks or months will show clearly any changes which are taking place, and whether any trend is up or down.

5.2 The Arithmetic Mean — Ungrouped Data

Table 5.1 shows the number of beds occupied each day of a week for a ward of 40 beds. The bed-occupancy rate is the number of beds divided by 40.

The mean number of beds occupied per day is:

$$\frac{39 + 40 + 39 + 37 + 36 + 34 + 38}{7} = \frac{263}{7}$$

$$= 37.57 \text{ beds}$$

Table 5.1 Bed-occupancy in Ward A

Day	Number of beds occupied	Bed-occupancy rate
Monday	39	0.975
Tuesday	40	1.000
Wednesday	39	0.975
Thursday	37	0.925
Friday	36	0.900
Saturday	34	0.850
Sunday	38	0.950

If a mean bed-occupancy rate is required, divide 37.57 by 40 to get 0.939. This could also have been obtained as a mean derived from the daily bed-occupancy rates.

Note. We will now introduce algebraic notation which is a convenient and universal shorthand way of stating what we are doing.

$\bar{x}$ (pronounced x-bar) = arithmetic mean

x_i (pronounced x-i) = representative value of a variable

n = total number of items

Σ (pronounced sigma) = sum of items following

The formal expression for the arithmetic mean is

$$\text{Arithmetic Mean } (\bar{x}) = \frac{\sum_{i=1}^{n} x_i}{n}$$

The subscript and superscript attached to Σ give the range of values of x_i; these are $x_1, x_2, x_3, \ldots, x_n$, the n individual values of the variable.

There are seven values of the variable, number of occupied beds per day. So these are expressed algebraically as $x_1, x_2, \ldots, x_6, x_7$. The expression for the mean can be given limits indicating seven values and then expanded:

$$\bar{x} = \frac{\sum_{i=1}^{7} x_i}{7} = \frac{x_1 + x_2 + x_3 + x_4 + x_5 + x_6 + x_7}{7}$$

To complete the calculation, we would insert the values of x from the data.

Calculating the mean in this way is simple where there are only a few values, but is time consuming for large data sets. This is easily overcome using a computer and suitable software. Otherwise, a common solution to handling large numbers of items is to group them first into like categories before calculating the mean (see section 5.3 following).

A warning. Watch out for extreme values in a data set—either very high or very low values. These can distort the mean, especially if the total number of values is not large, or if the extreme values are a notable percentage of all values. A mean distorted in this way could be quite unrepresentative of the data, and therefore not at all useful.

An example. Suppose a group of 25 patients suffering from a particular complaint are being studied to see how long treatment was continued before they recovered. Here are the number of days' treatment for the patients:

Table 5.2 Number of days' treatment per patient

3	4	5	7	8
3	5	6	7	8
4	5	6	7	21
4	5	6	7	36
4	5	6	8	45

The mean number of days' treatment for these 25 patients is 9 days. This does not in any real sense describe the original data. Of the 25 patients, 22 show periods of treatment within a narrow range, 3 to 8 days, but 3 cases are maverick: 21, 36 and 45 days respectively. Common sense tells us that in these 3 cases, long term treatment is likely to reflect special circumstances and that these may not be comparable to the other 22 cases. We must review the criteria by which we are conducting the study. Should all cases be taken together? If so, a mean period of treatment will have little significance. Are there other factors possibly affecting length of treatment by which cases should be divided into separately analysed subgroups? This raises important questions of research design (see Chapter 9).

5.3   The Arithmetic Mean—Grouped Data

An arithmetic mean can be calculated from grouped data. Each separate value of the variable (x) that occurs is multiplied by its frequency (f), the number of times it occurs, the products (xf)* totalled and this total divided by the total number of items (n). The data on age of hospital dental staff in Table 5.3 do not show individual ages but the number of staff whose age comes within each of several 5 and 10 year age-groups, plus two open-ended age-groups.

In calculating the arithmetic mean we use the class midpoint, midway between the lowest and highest values (class limits) as the age which

---

* If in an algebraic expression two variables are placed together, for example xf, this means they are multiplied together.

Table 5.3   Age of hospital dental staff at 30 September 1987*

Age in years	Number of staff
Under 30	398
30 and under 35	123
35 and under 40	120
40 and under 50	289
50 and under 60	220
60 and under 65	77
65 and over	8
All ages	1,235

* Staff holding permanent paid (whole-time and part-time) and/or
honorary appointments in the NHS Hospital Service.
Source: DH (1989) *Health and Personal Social Services Statistics
for England 1989*, HMSO.

'represents' the age of all hospital dental staff whose age falls in that class.
So for those 30 and under 35 years the midpoint is 32.5 years; for 35 and
under 40 years the midpoint is 37.5 years; for 40 and under 50 years it is
45.0 years.[†]

Now to the problem of the open-ended classes. The aim is to pick a value
which itself reasonably reflects the mean of the age composition of these
groups. The decision matters more where the group is large (398 dental staff
under the age of 30 years) rather than small (8 in the age-group 65 years and
over). Amongst those under 30 years, some will be under 25 years but on
account of the length of their training, the majority will be above this age.
As a 'representative' value, 27.5 years could be reasonable to use (midpoint
25 and under 30 years). We might select a higher age, say 28.0 or 28.5 years
if we think many might be close to 30 years, or a lower age, 27.0
or 26.5 years, if we anticipated a large group under 25 years. In the absence
of more information, we will use 27.5 years. There are very few dentists
aged 65 years and over (8—less than 1% of the total). A representative value
of 67.5 years is convenient, the midpoint of 65 and under 70 years. We
should not choose a higher value, but could reasonably select a lower one.
Whatever is chosen will have a minimal effect on the mean.

To calculate the mean, the number of hospital dental staff in each age-
group is multiplied by the midpoint value; these products are summed, and
then divided by the total number of staff. In the calculation in Table 5.4,

---

[†] Note that '30 and under 35 years' is treated as if it were '30–35 years', with midpoint 32.5,
and similarly for the other age-groups. This is because the age-group '30 and under 35 years'
will include all in age from those who are exactly 30 years on 30 September 1987, to those who
will be 35 years on 1 October 1987. For all practical purposes, this means 30–35 years.
(Try working out 34 years 364 days to two decimal places: it is 35.00.) Age data expressed
in classes as 30–34, 35–39, 40–49 years etc., should be treated as 30 and under 35, 35 and under
40, 40 and under 50 years etc., with midpoints 32.5 years, 37.5 years, 45 years etc.

columns 1 and 2 contain the original information on age range and number of staff; column 3 shows the midpoints and column 4 the result of multiplying the age midpoints (column 3) by the number of staff (column 2). We also need total frequency (column 2) and the sum of the products (column 4).

Table 5.4 Age of hospital dental staff, 1987

(1) Age in years	(2) No. of staff (f)	(3) Midpoints (x)	(4) col(3) × col(2) ($x \times f = xf$)
Under 30	398	27.5	10,945
30 and under 35	123	32.5	3,997.5
35 and under 40	120	37.5	4,500
40 and under 50	289	45	13,005
50 and under 60	220	55	12,100
60 and under 65	77	62.5	4,812.5
65 and over	8	67.5	540
	$n = 1,235$*		$\sum xf = 49,900$

* Note that n is the same as $\sum f$, the sum of the frequencies. The convention in statistical formulae is to use n rather than $\sum f$ to represent total frequency, total number of items.

$$\bar{x} = \frac{\sum xf}{n} = \frac{49,900}{1,235} = 40.40 \text{ years}$$

Note. The formula used in this calculation is

$$\bar{x} = \frac{\sum_{i=1}^{k} x_i f_i}{n}$$

Expanding this in terms of the example above:

$$\bar{x} = \frac{x_1 f_1 + x_2 f_2 + x_3 f_3 + x_4 f_4 + x_5 f_5 + x_6 f_6 + x_7 f_7}{n}$$

$$= \frac{27.5 \times 398 + 32.5 \times 123 + \cdots + 62.5 \times 77 + 67.5 \times 8}{1,235}$$

$$= \frac{49,900}{1,235} = 40.40 \text{ years}$$

5.4 The Weighted Mean

If a large group is divided into subgroups (for example, patients in wards), and the arithmetic mean for each subgroup (length of in-patient stay) is known, this can be used to calculate the mean for the group as a whole.

For each of four wards, the mean length of stay has been calculated over a period of three months.

Table 5.5 Length of in-patient stay

(1) Ward	(2) No. of patients discharged	(3) Mean in-patient stay (days)	(4) col(2) × col(1)
A	260	7.2	1,872
B	180	9.1	1,638
C	210	8.6	1,806
D	130	10.3	1,339
Totals	780		6,655

$$\bar{x} = \frac{6,655}{780} = 8.5 \text{ days}$$

To obtain the overall mean, the mean length of stay in each ward (column 3) is multiplied by the number of patients discharged (column 2), providing the total number of in-patient days for the patients discharged from that ward, the result being entered in column (4). Adding together these products gives the total number of in-patient days for the patients from all four wards, and dividing by total patients gives the arithmetic mean.* This is called the weighted mean because the mean length of in-patient stay for each ward has been 'weighted' by the number of patients discharged.

A reminder. Much of the data comes in whole numbers—patients, beds, nurses, out-patient clinics, prescriptions dispensed, meals served. Calculated measures based on whole numbers are not so restricted and, if justified by the data, are legitimately calculated to one or more decimal places. Look at *Health and Personal Social Services Statistics for England* for examples.

There is a general point at issue here. The accuracy used must reflect both the magnitude of the original data and the use to which the computed measures are to be put. Do they need to be very accurate? For comparative purposes? For further use, perhaps in more computations? Or will reasonably rounded figures do? Think about the level of accuracy in relation to all calculated measures, not only in respect of central values.

---

* Do not add together the mean in-patient stay for each of the four wards and divide by four. This does not allow for the different numbers of patients discharged from each ward, and would give a wrong answer.

5.5 The Median — Ungrouped Data

The median is another average in common use. It is the middle value of a data set, with half the values above the median, half below. The figures for daily bed-occupancy (Table 5.1) can be arranged in descending order:

Table 5.6 Bed-occupancy in Ward A

Day	Occupied beds
Tuesday	40
Monday	39
Wednesday	39
Sunday	38
Thursday	37
Friday	36
Saturday	34

Since there are an odd number of values (7), the fourth, which is 38 beds, is the median. If there are an even number of values, then the median is taken as midway (the mean) between the two middle values. Consider the following monthly figures for mean bed-occupancy in a ward:

Table 5.7 Bed-occupancy in Ward A

Month	Mean bed-occupancy	Month	Mean bed occupancy	Month	Mean bed-occupancy
Jan	39.5	May	37.9	Sept	37.4
Feb	38.4	June	36.4	Oct	38.3
March	38.8	July	36.2	Nov	38.5
April	37.3	August	37.8	Dec	39.2

Arranged in descending order these are:

Table 5.8 Bed-occupancy in Ward A

Month	Mean bed-occupancy	Month	Mean bed-occupancy	Month	Mean bed-occupancy
Jan	39.5	Feb	38.4	Sept	37.4
Dec	39.2	Oct	38.3	April	37.3
March	38.8	May	37.9	June	36.4
Nov	38.5	August	37.8	July	36.2

The two middle values in sixth and seventh places are October (38.3 beds), and May (37.9 beds), with midpoint 38.1 beds. This is the median.

For a small number of items, it is easy to find the middle value(s); not so with a large data set. A computer experiences no such problems, simply ordering the data in the same way as we have done, and then selecting the middle value as the median. With a large data set the data may be grouped for ease of handling, so the next step is to calculate the median with grouped data.

5.6   The Median — Grouped Data

Exactly the same principle operates as for ungrouped data; the median is the middle value of the grouped data, dividing total frequency into two equal parts. The data on the age of hospital dental staff (Table 5.3) is shown as a histogram in Figure 5.1.

There are 1,235 dentists, half total frequency is 617.5* and the median has been drawn on the histogram with 617.5 frequency either side of it. The median age lies somewhere between 35 and 40 years. How do we find where it lies? Look at the information on the age of hospital dental staff like this:

There are 398 dentists under 30 years of age.

There are 398 + 123 (= 521) dentists under 35 years of age.

There are 521 + 120 (= 641) dentists under 40 years of age.

So frequency 617.5, pinpointing the median value, must lie somewhere between 35 and 40 years. This is known as the median class.

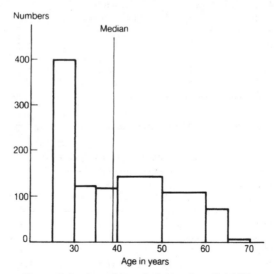

Figure 5.1   Age of hospital dental staff 1987

* Using a frequency including a fraction of a dentist is acceptable. This is a situation similar to the mean bed-occupancy calculation in section 2.

The point at which the median is located within the median class is obtained by dividing the class interval (5 years) in proportion to the number of dentists needed to reach the median frequency of 617.5. There are 521 dentists up to the bottom value of the median class (35 years) so another 96.5 (617.5 − 521) are needed to reach the median frequency of 617.5. This number (96.5) is divided by the number of dentists in the median class (120), then multiplied by the class interval. The calculation is as follows:

$$\text{Median} = 35 + \frac{96.5}{120} \times 5$$

$$= 35 + 0.804 \times 5$$

$$= 35 + 4.02 \text{ years} = 39.2 \text{ years, rounded to 39.0 years.}$$

Let us look at this a little more formally. When working out the number of dentists under 30 years of age, under 35 years, under 40 years, we created what is called a cumulative frequency distribution, a good starting point for calculating the median. Table 5.9 shows the data on age of hospital dental staff in its original form and as a cumulative frequency distribution.

Table 5.9   Age of hospital dental staff 1987

(1) Age in years	(2) Number of staff	(3) Cumulative frequency*	
Under 30	398	398	
30 and under 35	123	521	—number of dentists up to median class
35 and under 40 (median class)	120	641	—first cumulative frequency exceeding median frequency
40 and under 50	289	930	
50 and under 60	220	1,150	
60 and under 65	77	1,227	
65 and over	8	1,235	
All ages	1,235		

* Cumulative frequencies reflect the total number of dentists to the *upper* value of each class.

Here are the necessary steps in the calculation:

1. Median frequency $= \dfrac{\text{Total frequency}}{2} = \dfrac{1,235}{2} = 617.5$

2. First cumulative frequency to exceed 617.5 (641) is at age 40 years; the median class is 35 and under 40 years.

3. Up to age 35 years, cumulative frequency is 521; a further frequency of 96.5 (617.5 − 521) is required in the median class to reach the target frequency for the median of 617.5.

4. There are 120 dentists in the median class.

5. The median class interval is 5 years.

The calculation is exactly the same as before:

$$\text{Median} = 35 + \frac{96.5}{120} \times 5 = 39.02 \text{ years}$$

Note. There is no easy formula or expression for the median, and using notation as shorthand leads to the problem of needing to know and remembering how to interpret the notation. We can use the following formal expression:

$$\text{Median} = L_m + \frac{B_m \times C_m}{F_m}$$

where L_m = lower value of median class *

B_m = balance of frequency in median class to reach target frequency for median

F_m = frequency of median class—the number of items it contains

C_m = class interval of median class.

These values are from the original data and from the cumulative frequency distribution; the calculation itself is quite straightforward. Be careful to remember the basic idea behind the calculation and not to confuse the different meanings used in the expression.

An alternative. For those who are neat-fingered, the median can be obtained graphically. Cumulative frequencies are plotted on the vertical axis against the values of the variable age to which they relate (that is, against the upper values of each class) on the horizontal axis. Using the hospital dental staff data, we would plot the following points.

Table 5.10   Age of hospital dental staff 1987: cumulative frequencies

Vertical axis (cum. freq.)	398	521	641	930	1,150	1,227	1,235
Horizontal axis (age in years)	30	35	40	50	60	65	70

The resultant graph, called an ogive, is shown in Figure 5.2.

To complete the ogive we need to plot values representing the minimum and maximum ages for the hospital dentists. What have been used are the lower and upper values (class boundaries) implied by the 'midpoints' we selected when calculating the mean (section 3 above). The midpoints were

---

* This is the lower class boundary, see Chapter 2.5.

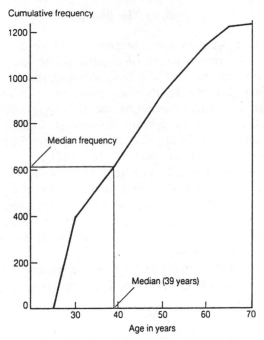

Figure 5.2 Age of hospital dental staff 1987

27.5 years and 65 years; the lower and upper class boundaries respectively were 25 years and 70 years. These values therefore have been used to complete the ogive.

Since the frequencies on the vertical axis are cumulative, this scale can be used to obtain the median. Select the point on the vertical scale corresponding to the median frequency (617.5). Use a ruler held horizontally to find the point on the ogive corresponding to the median frequency. Now take the ruler vertically from this point on the ogive, and find the corresponding value on the horizontal scale (age in years). This is the median age of hospital dentists.

A warning. The median tends to be more varied and less stable than the mean. The calculation of the mean takes account of all values but the median is determined only by the middle value(s) of the data. So if the middle value is in some way maverick, the median will be unreliable as a central measure. This is least likely to be the case where the total frequency is large. On the other hand, an advantage of the median is that unlike the mean, it is unaffected by extreme values. The median is descriptive, providing a value midway through total frequency. Unlike the mean, the median cannot enter into further calculations because it lacks a mathematical relationship with all the data.

5.7 The Mode

The mode is the most commonly occurring value or characteristic in the data. If the most common length of in-patient stay in a hospital ward is 6 days, then an in-patient stay of 6 days would be the mode.

In a frequency distribution, the class containing the highest number is the modal class. In the distribution by age of hospital dentists, the modal class is under 30 years, since it contains the highest number of dentists, 398. Note that this shows clearly on the histogram (Figure 5.1).

A manufacturer of hospital equipment and supplies would be interested in the most commonly used size of an item, and this size would be the mode. (A phenomenon seen in chain stores selling clothes; sometimes we are all 'medium'.) Or another example: if different dressings are being tried out, and users asked to report their preferences, assessing overall ease of use, protective effect, outcome of use etc., the most commonly preferred dressing is the modal preference.

The mode, modal class and modal preference, are easy to understand but are seldom of practical interest or use. They are likely to appear only in a descriptive context.

5.8 The Three Central Measures

With data which forms a totally symmetrical distribution as in Figure 5.3 below, the mean, median and mode are identical at the centre of the distribution.

Data do not come in tidy symmetrical forms; rather distributions are skewed, more commonly positively than negatively. Positively skewed

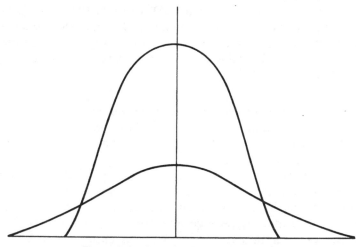

Figure 5.3 Symmetrical distributions

distributions have proportionately more dispersed higher values, negatively skewed distributions more dispersed lower values. In a positively skewed distribution, the mean always exceeds the median, which in its turn exceeds the mode, as in Figure 5.4a. In a negatively skewed distribution, the order is reversed—the mean is less than the median, which is less than the mode, as in Figure 5.4b.

For considered thought. Central measures are related to their data in ways which are individual to the particular measure. Which central measure to use? It depends on the intended purpose. Not usually the mode, unless we are interested only in general description. The mean or the median? A simple rule of thumb is 'the mean unless there is a good reason to the contrary.' Unless we are interested in the relationship of frequency to values of the variable (for example, that half the hospital dentists are under 39.0 years of age), we will choose the mean.

Both mean and median can be referred to as 'averages'. What do you make of those arguments rehearsed in wage negotiations when one party says '. . . and the average weekly earnings are £x . . .' to be countered by '. . . not so, average weekly earnings are £y . . .'. Assuming there

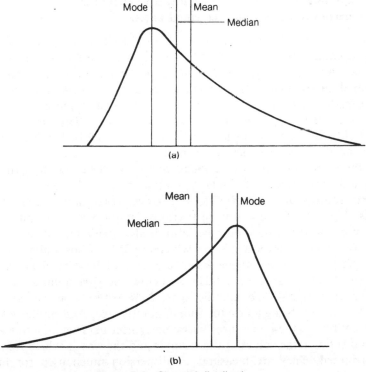

Figure 5.4 Skewed distributions

are no discrepancies in the definition of weekly earnings (net of national payments, holiday bonus, where is overtime? etc.) can both be right? (Earnings distributions are invariably positively skewed as in Figure 5.4a.)

5.9   The Quantiles

So far discussion has been of central measures. There are other measures, related to the median in that they divide frequency in specific ways. Strictly, they are measures of location or dispersion, not central measures, but their method of computation is the same as that for the median, and their relationship to the frequency distribution is a logical extension of that of the median. It is therefore practical to deal with them in this chapter rather than in the chapter following.

The median is central to the data, the value of the variable which divides total frequency into two equal parts. Other values are possible which divide the data in different ways, into whatever fractions desired. The measures commonly used are:

- three quartiles dividing frequency into four equal parts
- four quintiles dividing frequency into five equal parts
- nine deciles frequency into ten equal parts.

In addition there are ninety-nine percentiles dividing frequency into one hundred equal parts, but percentiles are in much less common use than quartiles, quintiles and deciles. The names of the individual measures reflect the way data are divided; the general name given to them all is Quantiles.

The median, as the name of a measure, takes precedence, so we never refer to the second quartile, the fifth decile or the fiftieth percentile. The same holds for other identical values; we refer to the first quintile not the second decile or the twentieth percentile.

As there are only two 'operational' quartiles, these may be termed the lower and upper quartiles. Similarly, we may refer to the lowest (first) and highest (fourth) quintiles, and to the lowest (first) and highest (ninth) deciles. Figures 5.5a, b and c, histograms for the age of hospital dental staff, show how quartiles, quintiles and deciles divide frequency.

The first quartile is the age below which are 25% of hospital dentists; the third quartile is the age above which are 25% of hospital dentists. With quintiles, think of 20% of dentists as below the first quintile age, 20% between first and second quintile ages, 20% between second and third quintiles, to 20% being above the fourth quintile age. And similarly for the deciles. Why are these measures particularly useful? They describe a relationship between the values of the variable and the way in which frequency is distributed. They are measures of dispersion much used for income and earnings distributions, wealth distributions and age distributions, and

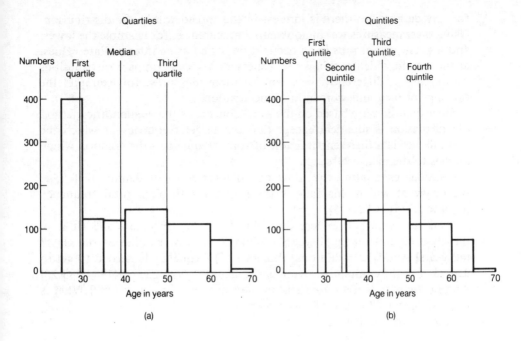

(a)

(b)

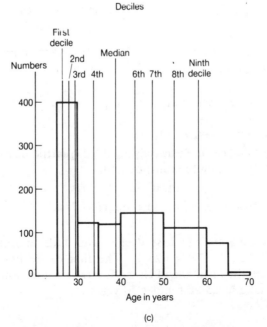

(c)

Figure 5.5 Age of hospital dental staff 1987

for any data where there is interest in the spread within the distribution. Using these measures we can look either at extremes, for example the lowest and highest paid groups in an occupation, or by using intermediate values, at the way in which earnings are dispersed. We can compare distributions by looking at differences between the same measures, for example, the earnings of men and women in an occupation.

Since quantiles are based on the same concept as the median, the method of calculation is identical except that the target frequency at which the quantile lies is a different fraction of total frequency—the fraction which applies to the measure sought.

Consider calculating the third quartile for hospital dental staff. The frequency at which this falls is three quarters through total frequency $[(3/4 \times 1{,}235) = 926.25]$.

Look at Table 5.9. Where does this frequency [926.25] fall? (It is in the class 40 and under 50 years.) What is the lower value of the class? [40 years] And what additional (balance of) frequency is needed to get to 926.25 after the cumulative frequency to age 40? $[(926.25 - 641) = 285.25]$ And how many dentists are there in the third quartile class? [289] What is the class interval? [40 to 50 = 10 years]

So the third quartile is:

$$40 + \frac{285.25}{282} \times 10 \text{ years} = 40 + 9.87$$

$$= 49.87 \text{ years, rounded to } 49.9 \text{ years.}$$

Note. We can produce a formal expression for the third quartile (or for any other quantile) analogous to that for the median:

$$Q_3 \text{ (third quartile)} = L_{Q_3} + \frac{B_{Q_3} \times C_{Q_3}}{F_{Q_3}}$$

where L_{Q_3} = lower value of Q_3 class

B_{Q_3} = balance of frequency in third quartile class to reach target frequency for third quartile

F_{Q_3} = frequency of third quartile class

C_{Q_3} = class interval of third quartile class.

Suppose we require the first decile. This falls at one tenth of total frequency $[(1/10 \times 1{,}235) = 123.5]$. The first decile lies within the first class, originally the open-ended class, 'under 30 years' which was closed at 25 years to make it '25 and under 30 years'.*

---

* Hence the practical need to close open-ended classes.

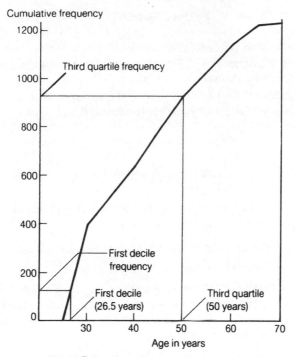

Figure 5.6 Age of hospital dental staff 1987

The calculation follows the same pattern—try it for yourself. The answer is included with answers to the questions at the end of this chapter.

Back to the ogive. The ogive can be used to obtain any of these measures by reading from the graph. Figure 5.6 shows the ogive (a repeat of Figure 5.2) but this time with the third quartile and the first decile. Try reading off some more measures for yourself, for example, the five quintiles.

5.10 Summary

You have learnt much in this chapter. You can now:

- define the arithmetic mean, and calculate it from both grouped and ungrouped data:
- define and calculate the median and any other of the related measures, the quantiles;
- draw an ogive and obtain the median and the quantiles graphically from it;
- identify the mode in a data set;
- make use of the mean, median and mode as appropriate central measures;
- use the quantiles as descriptive measures of dispersion.

Further Reading

For a useful discussion on central measures:
Freund J E and Williams F J (1970 2nd edn) *Modern Business Statistics*
  Chapter 3. London: Pitman.
A helpful comparison of the various central measures is in Blalock H M
  (1979 2nd edn) *Social Statistics* Chapter 5.4 and 5.5. Tokyo: McGraw-
  Hill Kogakusha.

A Little Practice

1. What is (a) the median and (b) the mode for the number of days
treatment per patient in Table 5.2?

2. Calculate the mean and the median for the data on the height of student
nurses (Chapter 2 question 1).

3. Now draw an ogive for the student nurse data. (Remember that upper
class boundaries are plotted against the cumulative frequencies.) Read off
the values for (a) the first and third quartiles; (b) the first and fourth
quintiles; and (c) the first and ninth deciles.

4. Using the data on the age of 35 patients (Chapter 3 question 2), calculate
(a) the mean, (b) the median and (c) the first and third quartiles. (Remember
to close the two open-ended classes before starting your computations.)

6

Measures of Dispersion: Standard Deviation and Others

6.1 The Range

Central measures provide single values which are in some way representative of all the data. This may not be sufficient in that we may wish to know something about the variation or dispersion or spread in data.

The range is the simplest measure of dispersion. It is the difference between the highest and lowest values in data. Take the data on number of days' treatment (Table 5.2). The highest value is 45 days, the lowest 3 days, so the range is 42. In this example the range is not very helpful because it is wide in relation to the generality of the data on account of the three extreme values (22 out of 25 lengths of stay are between 3 and 8 days). For the distribution by age of hospital dental staff (Table 5.3), the range would be 45 years, the difference between the lowest value of the lowest class (25) and the highest value of the highest class (70). Generally the range is of limited value, but it is simple and easy to calculate and may be helpful in giving a very broad view of the spread in the data.

6.2 Quantiles: The Interquartile Range and Others

The concept of the range can be extended to the measures related to the median. The difference between the lower (first) and upper (third) quartiles is called the interquartile range. For the hospital dental staff, the lower quartile is 28.9 years, the upper quartile 49.9 years, so the interquartile range is 21.0 years. This gives the spread in the age of the 'middle 50%' of hospital dentists. We could say that 'the middle 50% of hospital dentists are aged between 28.9 years and 49.9 years'. The interquartile range is less frequently referred to than the quartiles themselves, that 25% of frequency is below the lower quartile, 25% of frequency above the upper quartile.

Quintiles and deciles can be used similarly. We can look at changes in these values over time, or can use them to compare two distributions. A narrow 'middle range' of data indicates less variation than would a wide 'middle range'. More commonly, lowest and highest quintiles and deciles would be used to say, for example, of hospital dentists that the youngest 20% are aged under 28.1 years and the oldest 20% are aged above 52.6 years.*

6.3   The Standard Deviation

This is a very important measure of dispersion. It takes account of all the values in a data set, and is based on the difference between each value and the mean of the data. In definitional terms, the difference between each individual value and the mean of the data is squared; the squared differences added; their sum divided by total frequency to get a mean squared difference; and finally the square root taken to get back into linear measure.[†]

Let us calculate the standard deviation for the data on the number of days' treatment per patient (Table 5.2), for which the mean was 9 days ($\bar{x} = 9$). The initial calculation is in Table 6.1. Values of x represent the number of days' treatment per patient, $\bar{x}$ the mean number of days' treatment, and $(x - \bar{x})$ the difference between each individual value of x and the mean days of treatment. Finally the last difference is squared.

The calculation is completed by dividing the sum of the squared differences from the mean [$\sum (x - \bar{x})^2 = 2{,}476$] by the number of patients [$n = 25$] to obtain a mean squared difference [99.04]; the square root is the standard deviation of 9.95 days.

The standard deviation is high because of the effect of the three extreme values. This is quite clear in Table 6.1. Had the three extreme values been excluded, the mean length of stay for 22 patients would have been 5.59 days with standard deviation 1.53 days. This potential distortion by extreme values is most likely to occur if the data set is small (here 25 patients), and the extreme values form a notable percentage of total frequency (here 12%). With several hundred values of which few were extreme, say less than 1%, the possible distorting effect would be minimal.

---

* The New Earnings Survey, DE, is carried out annually and relates to earnings in April of each year. It is based on a simple random sample (see Chapter 7.1 and 7.2) which selects 1% of employees in Great Britain using National Insurance numbers. Returns on earnings are made by employers. The data is presented in various forms—by industry, occupation, broad categories of employment, region and by sex and age. Considerable use is made of quantiles of earnings. Upper and lower quartiles, and highest (ninth) and lowest (first) deciles are quoted as well as means (referred to as 'averages'), and medians. These make sharp points in looking comparatively at different distributions of earnings. See for example earnings patterns in nursing as between administrative and nursing/midwifery staff, and between men and women. (NES Tables 96 section III and 97 section III.)

[†] Why bother to square the differences, to add them, to find their mean, and finally to take a square root? Some of the differences from the mean will be positive (values greater than the mean) and some negative (values less than the mean). Their total will always be zero, as in the example following. Mathematically, squaring values disposes of the minus sign. More importantly, there is a fundamental mathematical basis for the measure.

Table 6.1 Number of days' treatment per patient

Days (x)	($x - \bar{x}$)	($x - \bar{x}$)^2	Days (x)	($x - \bar{x}$)	($x - \bar{x}$)^2
3	−6	36	6	−3	9
3	−6	36	6	−3	9
4	−5	25	7	−2	4
4	−5	25	7	−2	4
4	−5	25	7	−2	4
4	−5	25	7	−2	4
5	−4	16	8	−1	1
5	−4	16	8	−1	1
5	−4	16	8	−1	1
5	−4	16	21	+12	144
5	−4	16	36	+27	729
6	−3	9	45	+36	1,296
6	−3	9	Totals	$\sum (x - \bar{x}) = 0$	$\sum (x - \bar{x})^2 = 2{,}476$

Note. The formula used above to calculate the standard deviation (s) is:

$$s = \sqrt{\frac{\sum_{i=1}^{n} (x_i - \bar{x})^2}{n}}$$

and is the definitive formula, describing the standard deviation as a measure derived from the squared differences between the original data and their mean value. It is not a formula used to calculate this measure.

The calculation was quite straightforward using the definitive formula because the mean was a whole number—an exceptional circumstance. Differences were exact, squaring them easy. If the mean had not been a whole number, as when the extreme values were excluded, and the mean was approximately 5.59 days, the calculation would have been more difficult. And more difficult still had numbers of cases been larger. The standard deviation is never calculated this way. The formula used is set out and discussed in the **note** following.

Note. The operational formula for the standard deviation is:

$$s = \sqrt{\frac{\sum_{i=1}^{n} x_i^2}{n} - \frac{\left(\sum_{i=1}^{n} x_i\right)^2}{n}} \qquad \text{simplified to*}$$

$$s = \sqrt{\frac{\sum x^2}{n} - \left(\frac{\sum x}{n}\right)^2}$$

---

*In this and in the preceding chapter, formulae have been written with the limits of value for summations. This is to emphasise the meaning of these formulae. In the remainder of the book, limits of value will be ignored and formulae expressed in simplified form with limits of value implied.

where $\sum x_i^2$ is the sum of the squared values of x, the individual number of days' treatment; n is the total number of patients; $\sum x_i/n$ is the formula for the mean, the sum of the individual values of x divided by n the number of patients. In the standard deviation formula above, $\sum x/n$ is used rather than $\bar{x}$.

A warning. Be careful not to confuse $\sum x^2$, which is the sum of the squared values of x, with $(\sum x)^2$, which is the square of the sum of the values of x. The two are quite different, and $(\sum x)^2$ is always larger than $\sum x^2$. You can demonstrate this for yourself using the numbers 1, 2, 3 and 4 as values of x.

This formula is a mathematical rearrangement of the original definitive expression for the standard deviation. Easier to handle, it avoids calculating an inexact mean to obtain values of $(x - \bar{x})$, which will themselves be inexact. The formula relates to basic data values, and is the way a computer would calculate the standard deviation.

———

Let us repeat the calculation for the number of days' treatment using the new formula.

Table 6.2 Number of days' treatment per patient

Days (x)	x^2	Days (x)	x^2
3	9	6	36
3	9	6	36
4	16	7	49
4	16	7	49
4	16	7	49
4	16	7	49
5	25	8	64
5	25	8	64
5	25	8	64
5	25	21	441
5	25	36	1,296
6	36	45	2,025
6	36		
		Totals $\sum x = 225$	$\sum x^2 = 4{,}501$

Using the rearranged formula:

$$s = \sqrt{\frac{4{,}501}{25} - \left(\frac{225}{25}\right)^2} = \sqrt{180.04 - 81} = \sqrt{99.04}$$

$$= 9.95 \text{ days}$$

the same as for the earlier calculation.

6.4   The Standard Deviation—Grouped Data

However large the data set, a computer will handle the calculation of the standard deviation by the method just used. What is also required is a method of calculating the standard deviation for grouped data. Rearranging the data on in-patient stay by grouping together those with the same length of stay produces a frequency distribution. To calculate the standard deviation allowing for the frequency with which each value occurs, we *weight* the values of x and x^2 by the number of times each value of x occurs. The rearranged data and the calculation are shown in Table 6.3

Table 6.3   Number of days' treatment per patient

(1) Days (x)	(2) Number of patients (f)	(3) col(1) × col(2) ($x \times f = xf$)	(4) col(1) × col(3) ($x \times xf = x^2f$)
3	2	6	18
4	4	16	64
5	5	25	125
6	4	24	144
7	4	28	196
8	3	24	192
21	1	21	441
36	1	36	1,296
45	1	45	2,025
	$n = 25$	$\sum xf = 225$	$\sum x^2f = 4,501$

Note: to get values of x^2f, multiply values from col(1), x, by those from col(3), xf. Be careful not to use col(2), f, the frequency, instead of col(1), x.

The values of x are no longer the individual number of days of treatment, but the different lengths of treatment. Multiplying number of days of treatment (x) by number of patients with that length of treatment (f), gives exactly the same result with total $\sum xf$ as $\sum x$ in the earlier calculation using the individual lengths of treatment. $\sum x^2f$ is the same as the 'sum of squared values of x', $\sum x^2$. We would use these totals ($\sum xf$, $\sum x^2f$) in exactly the same way as the earlier totals ($\sum x$, $\sum x^2$) and get the same value for the standard deviation. The final calculation is an exact repeat of that at the end of section 3 above.

A point. The calculation above produces the mean ($\sum xf/n$) as well as the standard deviation. This is useful because the two measures are commonly required together.

Note. The formula just used is:

$$s = \sqrt{\frac{\sum x^2 f}{n} - \left(\frac{\sum xf}{n}\right)^2}$$

A warning. Be careful to interpret this correctly. $\sum x^2 f$ is the sum of the squared values which have been 'weighted' by frequency. The frequencies are not squared. $\sum xf$ is the sum of the individual values, weighted by frequency.

Now to calculate the standard deviation for the age of hospital dental staff using the data from Chapter 5.

Table 6.4 Age of hospital dental staff 1987

(1) Age in years	(2) Number of dentists (f)	(3) Age mid-points (x)	(4) col(3) × col(2) ($x \times f = xf$)	(5) col(3) × col(4) ($x \times xf = x^2 f$)
under 30	398	27.5	10,945	300,987.5
30 and under 35	123	32.5	3,997.5	129,918.75
35 and under 40	120	37.5	4,500	168,750
40 and under 50	289	45	13,005	585,225
50 and under 60	220	55	12,100	665,500
60 and under 65	77	62.5	4,812.5	300,781.25
65 and over	8	67.5	540	36,450
	$n = 1,235$		$\sum xf = 49,900$	$\sum x^2 f = 2,187,612.50$

Inserting the summations in the formula:

$$s = \sqrt{\frac{\sum x^2 f}{n} - \left(\frac{\sum xf}{n}\right)^2}$$

$$= \sqrt{\frac{2,187,612.5}{1,235} - \left(\frac{49,900}{1,235}\right)^2}$$

$$= \sqrt{1,771.35 - (\underline{\underline{40.405}})^2}$$

$$= \sqrt{1,771.35 - 1,632.56}$$

$$= \sqrt{138.79}$$

$$= 11.78 \text{ years}$$

The mean was calculated (see double underlining above) as 40.05 years.

The calculation is straightforward despite the rather large numbers in col(5).

Contemplation. What meaning has the standard deviation? What is it used for? The standard deviation is a measure of dispersion or variation; it is related to all the data—each and every item enters into the calculation. It is mathematically derived so it can enter into further calculations and relate to other measures. It is essential in Part III following.

A comment. We noted that the mean was affected by extreme values, and so is the standard deviation—even more so. When the three extreme values from the hospital in-patients are excluded, leaving 22 patients, the mean number of days' treatment is 5.59 days with standard deviation 1.53 days, very different values from those calculated from all 25 patients, a mean of 9.00 days and a standard deviation of 9.95 days.

Looking at the hospital dentists, very few are aged 65 years and over (8—just more than half of 1% of frequency). If excluded, what would be the effect on the mean and standard deviation? The answer is very little; the mean would be 40.23 years instead of 40.40 years, and the standard deviation would be 11.61 years instead of 11.78 years. These differences are marginal because the extreme values are such a small proportion of total frequency.

For thought. What is a small data set? Information is lost when data are grouped into classes because instead of original values, the midpoints of the classes are used as the 'representative value' for each class. The loss of information by grouping is reduced as the total number of items increases. The larger the data set, the closer the mean and standard deviation of grouped data will be to the exact measures obtained by using the original values. It would be unwise (for calculation purposes) to group fewer than 100 items into classes, safer to group data where there were at least 300 values. This emphasises the advantages of using a computer which will produce exact measures.

6.5 The Coefficient of Variation

We may need to compare the dispersion in two distributions, for example, to decide whether there is more variation in length of in-patient stay of dermatology patients than of infectious diseases patients (or vice versa). For dermatology patients the mean length of in-patient stay is 19.7 days with standard deviation 3.5 days; for infectious diseases patients, the mean length of in-patient stay is 7.5 days with standard deviation 2.0 days. Do not leap to the conclusion that because the standard deviation for dermatology patients' length of stay is nearly twice that for infectious diseases patients, there is greater variation in the dermatology patients' length of stay.

Proper comparison is through the coefficient of variation. This expresses the standard deviation as a percentage of the mean:

$$\text{coefficient of variation} = \frac{s}{\bar{x}} \times 100$$

For the two groups of patients:

Dermatology patients

$$\text{coefficient of variation} \quad = \frac{3.5}{19.7} \times 100$$

$$= 17.8$$

Infectious diseases patients

$$\text{coefficient of variation} \quad = \frac{2.0}{7.5} \times 100$$

$$= 26.7$$

The conclusion from this is that the length of in-patient stay of infectious diseases patients is more varied than the length of in-patient stay for dermatology patients.

The coefficient of variation is a ratio and therefore permits comparison of distributions where orders of magnitude are different (as in this example) and also where different units of measurement are involved.

6.6   The Variance

The variance is the square of the standard deviation (s^2). It has no conceptual meaning since there are no squared days (length of in-patient stay) or squared years (age of hospital dental staff) etc. It is another way of looking at the variation or dispersion in the data, and we shall come across it again in Chapters 14 and 16.

6.7   Summary

In this chapter we have learnt to:

- define the range, and understand measures of dispersion drawn from the quantiles, and the standard deviation as the mathematical measure of dispersion;
- calculate the standard deviation, from both ungrouped and grouped data;
- define and calculate the coefficient of variation and the variance.

Further Reading

A broader discussion of measures of dispersion is to be found in:
Freund J E and Williams F J (1970 2nd edn) *Modern Business Statistics*
  Chapter 4. London: Pitman.

A Little Practice

1. Using the data on the height of student nurses (Chapter 2 question 1) calculate the standard deviation of the mean.

2. Using the data on number of out-patients visits (Chapter 2 question 3), calculate the mean and the standard deviation.

3. Using the data on the age of 35 patients (Chapter 3 question 2), calculate the standard deviation.

4. Length of in-patient stay:

Number of days (x)	Number of patients (f)
3	12
4	47
5	68
6	34
7	16
8 to 10	11
over 10	6
All patients	194

Calculate the mean and standard deviation for the above data on the length of in-patient stay for patients undergoing a particular surgical procedure. (Note: the single values, 3, 4 etc. behave as the midpoints of classes. You need a midpoint for the class 8 to 10 days, and must choose a suitable representative value for the class 'over 10 days'.)

Part III

Statistical Inference

7

The Preliminaries to Sampling Theory

7.1 The Population and the Sample

Population: also called universe. Statistics: the entire finite or infinite aggregate of individuals or items from which samples are drawn.

Sample: a small part of anything, intended as representative of the whole.

Collins English Dictionary (1991 3rd edn).

The following chapters of Part III are concerned with drawing conclusions from samples. Understanding about sampling and about samples is therefore essential since most research is based on samples. If we are investigating the outcomes of a particular treatment for a specific medical condition, we cannot study every patient (the population) who receives that treatment, but only some of them (a sample). If we draw samples in a particular way, the conclusions can apply to the whole population, apply not with certainty but with degrees of probability. To achieve this requires a framework, a theory, which relates a sample to its parent population.

Since a population consists of all the individuals or units in a group, the population to be sampled must be clearly defined. Populations can themselves be sub-populations of wider populations. For example, all patients in a particular NHS hospital are a population; they are also a sub-population of all patients in all NHS hospitals.

When studying the outcome of treatment given to hospital in-patients for a particular condition, we must not apply the findings of the study to a different group, for example those in the population of patients at large suffering from this condition. The hospital in-patients would be likely to be much more seriously affected than those not requiring in-patient treatment; the two groups are unlikely to be similar.

Before drawing a sample, we must define the population to which it relates, and ensure that the sample is drawn from that population and none other. Conclusions can only be drawn in respect of the particular population sampled.

Algebraic Notation—Sample and Population

In algebraic formulae it is necessary to distinguish between sample and population. There is an important convention that we refer to population parameters, using Greek letters to represent them, and to sample statistics, denoted by Roman letters. The most important measures for which these distinctions are needed are the mean and standard deviation. The population mean is represented by μ (pronounced 'mew'), the population standard deviation by σ (pronounced 'sigma'). For the sample, the mean is $\bar{x}$, and the standard deviation s as used already in Chapters 5 and 6.

7.2   Random Sampling

Random: Lacking any definite plan or prearranged order.
Collins English Dictionary (1991 3rd edn).

Where conclusions are to be drawn about the population from which the sample is drawn, samples must be random. The selection of sample units is left to chance—without bias, uninfluenced by subjective judgement. Every item in the population must have an opportunity of being included in the sample. In formal terms—every unit in the population must have a known, non-zero probability of selection and therefore of inclusion in the sample.*
A particular case is simple random sampling when each unit in the population has an equal chance of being included in the sample.

  The discussions on the theory of samples and sampling in section 4 following and the remainder of this chapter are based on simple random samples. In Chapter 9 we look at the practice; how samples may be drawn, how structured, what reasonably can be looked upon as a random sample. Meanwhile, a little theory.

7.3   Probability

Probability: 1. The condition of being probable. 2. An event or other thing that is probable. 3. Statistics: a measure or estimate of the degree of confidence one may have in the occurrence of an event, measured on a scale from zero (impossibility) to one (certainty). It may be defined as the proportion of favourable outcomes to the total number of possibilities if these are indifferent (mathematical probability), or the proportion observed in a sample (empirical probability).
Collins English Dictionary (1991 3rd edn).

---

*Sampling in this context is also referred to as probability sampling. If a sample is random, in the sense in which we are using that word, the inclusion of any item in a sample is subject to the rules of probability. Hence the term 'probability sampling' which is often used in this context.

To discover what happens when samples are selected randomly requires an understanding of probability. Instinctively, we all know something about probability—whether in terms of what happens when tossing coins or rolling dice, or the likelihood of being run down by a motor vehicle if crossing streets oblivious of the traffic.

We take total probability to be one. If out of a series of events one of them must happen, and a probability is assigned to each event, these probabilities add up to one. For a single event, the probability must lie between zero (it can never happen) and one (it must, like death, happen—certainty.)

We have a balanced die. When rolled, one of the faces will appear uppermost. There are six possible outcomes; if one occurs, another cannot. The outcomes are therefore termed 'mutually exclusive events'. Since the die is balanced, each face has the same probability of appearing uppermost—1/6.

Suppose we want the uppermost face to be a 5 or 6. The probability of a 5 appearing is 1/6, and of a 6 appearing is 1/6. So the probability of a 5 or a 6 appearing is [1/6 + 1/6 = 1/3]. This illustrates the first rule of probability, namely:

Rule 1:   The probability of two or more of a number of mutually exclusive events occurring is the sum of their separate probabilities.

(What would be the probability of a 4 or a 5 or a 6 appearing?)

Back to the die. What is the probability of rolling it twice and getting a six both times? Each roll of the die is independent of any other roll.* Since the probability of a six appearing on the first roll is 1/6, and 1/6 on the second roll, the probability of both rolls producing a 6 is [1/6 × 1/6 = 1/36]. This leads to the second rule of probability.

Rule 2:   The probability of two or more independent events both happening is the product of their separate probabilities.

(What would be the probability of three successive rolls all producing sixes? And four rolls?)

Events are not always mutually exclusive. If rolling a die twice to get at least one six (on either or both rolls), we cannot simply add the probabilities of getting a six on each roll [1/6 + 1/6 = 1/3]. This ignores the probability that two sixes are rolled [1/6 × 1/6]. For events which are not mutually exclusive, there is a different rule of addition.

---

* Sometimes this is difficult to believe. If tossing a balanced coin for heads results in a run of, say, six tails, it does not follow that the next toss is more likely to produce a head than a tail. The seventh toss is equally likely to produce a head as a tail.

Rule 3: If two events are not mutually exclusive, the probability that at least one occurs is the sum of their separate probabilities minus the probability that both occur (Rule 2—the product of their probabilities).

The probability of getting at least one six in two roles of a die is $[1/6 + 1/6 - (1/6 \times 1/6)]$ or 11/36.

Another important aspect of probability is conditional probability. Conditional probability is the probability that a second event will occur, provided a first event has already happened. The occurrence of the first event affects the probability of the second event occurring.

Consider this example. Following a particular surgical procedure, an 'unproblematic patient' is viewed as one whose temperature does not exceed 39°C 24 hours after the operation, and does not exceed 37°C 72 hours after the operation. From past patients' records, 70% achieve a temperature not exceeding 39°C within 24 hours (probability 0.7), and 80% achieve a temperature not exceeding 37°C within 72 hours (probability 0.8). What the records also show is that of patients who achieved the temperature of 39°C within 24 hours, 90% achieved a temperature of 37°C within 72 hours. The conditional probability that a patient's temperature will not exceed 37°C after 72 hours if the patient's temperature did not exceed 39°C after 24 hours is therefore 0.9. The probability of a patient being 'unproblematic' is therefore the probability that the patient's temperature does not exceed 39°C after 24 hours (0.7) multiplied by the conditional probability that having achieved this initial temperature, the patient's temperature does not exceed 37°C after 72 hours (0.9). The probability is 0.63. This leads to the fourth rule of probability:

Rule 4: The probability of two events which are not independent both happening is the probability that the first occurs multiplied by the conditional probability of the second occurring.

A last thought. A useful further way of looking at probability is to turn it round into the probability of something not happening. If the probability of an event happening is p, the probability of it not happening is $(1 - p)$. Rolling a die, the probability of not getting a six is the sum of the probabilities of all the other outcomes, which from Rule 1 is $[1/6 + 1/6 + 1/6 + 1/6 + 1/6 = 5/6]$. This is more easily obtained as $[1 - 1/6 = 5/6]$. Obvious, but a helpful way of thought we shall meet again.

7.4   The Binomial Distribution

Having learnt about randomness and probability, and using the probability rules of adding (Rule 1) and multiplying (Rule 2), we can consider a formal theoretical distribution called the Binomial Distribution.

If a balanced coin is tossed in an unbiased fashion (to obtain random samples), the coin is as likely to show a head uppermost as a tail. The probability of each of these outcomes is 1/2. Tossing four coins would result in any number of heads between 0 and 4 appearing uppermost but these 5 outcomes would not be equiprobable. To explore what happens when 4 coins are tossed together, look at all possible outcomes from tossing 4 coins in succession.

Table 7.1 Outcomes from tossing four coins

1st toss	2nd toss	3rd toss	4th toss
H	H	H	H
H	H	H	T
H	H	T	H
H	T	H	H
H	H	T	T
H	T	H	T
H	T	T	H
H	T	T	T
T	H	H	H
T	H	H	T
T	H	T	H
T	T	H	H
T	H	T	T
T	T	H	T
T	T	T	H
T	T	T	T

Allowing for the order in which heads and tails appeared, each outcome is different and each has a probability of 1/16 [Rule 2— $1/2 \times 1/2 \times 1/2 \times 1/2$]. To get the effect of tossing four coins together, ignore order; there are then five possible outcomes, the number of heads varying between 0 and 4. Adding probabilities (Rule 1) leads to Table 7.2.

Table 7.2 Outcomes from tossing four coins

Number of heads	Number of outcomes	Probability
0	1	1/16 or 0.0625
1	4	4/16 or 0.25
2	6	6/16 or 0.375
3	4	4/16 or 0.25
4	1	1/16 or 0.0625

[Note that total probability, obtained by adding the probabilities for the five separate outcomes, is 1.0.]

The histogram for this distribution is shown in Figure 7.1.

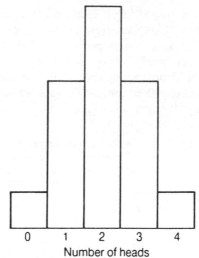

0   1   2   3   4
Number of heads

Figure 7.1   Outcomes from tossing four coins

The distribution of outcomes is symmetrical and the mean number of heads is 2. The most likely single result is also 2 heads [$p = 0.375$]. A result which differs by one from this, either 1 head or 3 heads [$p = 0.25 + 0.25 = 0.5$] has a higher probability. Either 0 or 4 heads is very much less likely.

As another example, consider tossing ten coins for heads. The outcomes and their probabilities are shown in Table 7.3, with the histogram in Figure 7.2.

Table 7.3   Outcomes from tossing ten coins

Number of heads	Probability
0	0.0010
1	0.0098
2	0.0439
3	0.1172
4	0.2051
5	0.2460
6	0.2051
7	0.1172
8	0.0439
9	0.0098
10	0.0010
	1.0000

Compare this ($n = 10$) with tossing 4 coins ($n = 4$). The mean number of heads is 5, but is a less likely outcome (probability = 0.2460) than getting

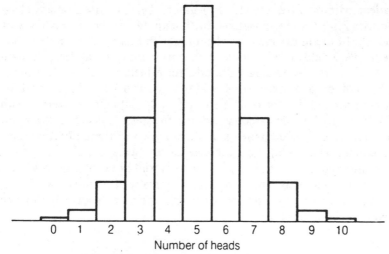

Number of heads

Figure 7.2   Outcomes from tossing ten coins

the mean number of heads when tossing 4 coins (probability = 0.375). Had we tossed 20 coins the mean number of heads would have been 10, but the probability of getting exactly 10 heads would have been less still—0.1762. The larger the sample size (n), the smaller the probability of a single result equalling the mean, but the greater the 'bunching' of the expected results round the mean.

This leads to the Binomial Distribution, which is the formal distribution demonstrated in these coin-tossing activities. It reflects the 'outcome' pattern of 'n trials' (coin-tossings) where p is the probability of 'success' (getting a head) in any one trial. The binomial distribution can be used to work out any pattern of outcomes where there is a known probability of success and a specific number of trials. If from previous records the probability of recovering without after-effects from a particular medical condition is known,* we can use that knowledge to investigate the results of a new piece of research.

Suppose out of a group of 60 patients suffering from a particular condition and experiencing a new treatment, 25 recover without after-effects. From previous records the probability of recovering without after-effects is 0.3. Out of 60 patients we would expect 18 to recover without after-effects [60 × 0.3]. How likely would be the outcome of the present study—25 out of 60 recovering fully? Using the binomial distribution is difficult because the probability of each outcome (no patient without after-effects,

---

*Records of patients would show how many, and therefore what proportion, recovered without after-effects. This proportion, a relative frequency, is the probability of recovering without after-effects.

1 patient without after-effects etc.) has to be computed separately—one thing if tossing 4 coins (5 outcomes), but quite another if dealing with 60 patients (61 outcomes) and overwhelming with really large numbers. For 60 patients we would have to look at the probability of at least 25 patients (i.e. 25 or more) recovering without after-effects as against less than this number (24 or less) recovering without after-effects. This requires the separate probabilities for 0, 1, 2 etc. up to 24 patients recovering without after-effects to be calculated, a tedious prospect.* What if the numbers were even larger—1,000 patients, and some two or three hundred separate calculations? The arithmetical exercise hardly bears thinking about.

The binomial distribution applies where a trial or event must result in one of two outcomes. Problems can often be arranged in this way. The basic principle is therefore of wide application; in practice the distribution used is the Normal Distribution.

Note. The formula for the Binomial Distribution[†] is

$$[p + (1 - p)]^n$$

where p is the probability of success in each trial, and n is the number of trials. Note the place of $(1 - p)$, the probability of 'failure'.

The mean of a binomial distribution is np (probability of 'success' multiplied by the number of trials). Its standard deviation is $\sqrt{np(1 - p)}$.

7.5   The Normal Distribution

The reason the binomial distribution is so awkward to use is that it is discrete, not continuous (see Chapter 2.5) and each frequency or probability has to be worked out separately for each discrete value. So we use another distribution, a continuous distribution known as the Normal Distribution. With a continuous distribution it is easy to obtain the relative frequency (probability) with which values occur in a particular range, that is, between two given values of a variable.

The origins of the normal distribution go back to Abraham de Moivre (1667–1745) and Carl Gauss (1777–1855). The former saw it as having application in games of chance (gambling was a great pastime for our fore-fathers in the seventeenth and eighteenth centuries), but Gauss developed

---

* That would be easier than calculating probabilities for 25, 26 etc. to 60 patients. We would add probabilities for 0 to 24 patients, and subtract the total from 1 to give the probability of 25 or more patients not suffering after-effects.
[†] The expansion of the binomial distribution is covered in many statistics textbooks.

it as a distribution of random errors. If a series of repeated measurements were taken, although the empirical measurements should be identical, there would be marginal variations and a pattern of errors would emerge. This pattern of errors approximated to a mathematical distribution, then known as the Normal Curve of Errors.

Later observation found that other data (for example the variable height, but much other simple numerical data as well) approximated to the bell-shaped distribution of the normal curve of errors. 'Errors' was dropped from its title and it became known as the 'normal distribution' or the 'normal curve'.

The binomial distribution, a discrete distribution, approximates closely to the continuous normal distribution with the same mean and standard deviation. Figure 7.3 shows binomial distributions overlaid with normal distributions.

Two things should be stressed. Firstly, the larger the value of n—the number of trials, the size of the sample—the more closely the binomial distribution approximates to the continuous normal distribution. For large values of n, the approximation is very close indeed. Secondly, the approximation is good for values of p other than $1/2$, and again the larger the value of n, the better the approximation.

If data approximate to the normal distribution, we may use the properties of that distribution to investigate and describe the data. In the research context, the pattern of measurements, such as arithmetic means, produced from a series of random samples (of the same size, drawn from the same

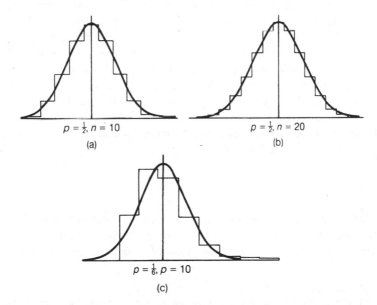

$p = \frac{1}{2}, n = 10$

(a)

$p = \frac{1}{2}, n = 20$

(b)

$p = \frac{1}{6}, p = 10$

(c)

Figure 7.3

population) approximates to the normal distribution. Hence the importance of the normal distribution in underpinning the sampling theory to be discussed in Chapter 8. Before reaching that point, we must establish a form of the normal distribution which can be used with any data.

7.6   The Standard Normal Distribution

We have examined the relationships between values of a variable (number of heads, number of sixes, number of patients who do not suffer after effects) and the relative frequency or probability with which particular values of the variable occur. Remember the histogram (Chapter 3.4); frequency was not represented by the height of the rectangular blocks but by their area. So too with the histograms from coin-tossing and die-rolling (Figure 7.3). The same applies to any continuous distribution of which the normal distribution is an example. The frequency with which values occur between two specific variable values, x_1 and x_2, is given by the proportion of the area under the continuous curve which lies between x_1 and x_2, as in Figure 7.4a and b.

When data approximate to the normal distribution, and we require particular areas to provide relative frequency or probability, the solution is the Standard Normal Distribution.

The mathematical formula for the normal distribution is formidable.* The crucial point is that the distribution is determined solely by its mean and standard deviation. Knowing these, we know everything about a particular normal distribution. Data which are approximately normally distributed have a variety of means and standard deviations. To simplify matters we substitute the standard normal distribution which has a mean of zero, a standard deviation of one and total frequency of one. Going back to original data (x), values can be converted into what is called 'standard form'. Values in standard form have a mean of zero, and a standard deviation of one. They are referred to as 'standard units' and are known as 'z' or 'z-values'. The transposition is:

$$z_i = \frac{x_i - \mu}{\sigma}$$

where μ is the mean, and σ the standard deviation of the original data and the value to be transposed into standard form is x_i. Figure 7.5 shows a normal distribution with the original 'x' scale and a 'z' scale.

———————————

*The formula for the normal distribution can be found in any standard statistics textbook.

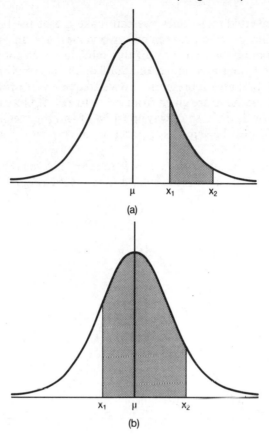

(a)

(b)

Figure 7.4

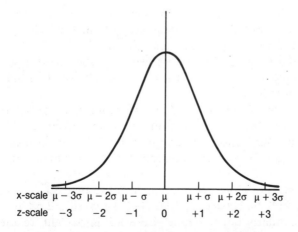

Figure 7.5

With data converted to z-values, we can make use of the Normal Curve
Area Table to find the area between any two values of z. In the Appendix,
Table 1 is the commonly used form of this table in which total area under
the curve equals 1, and area under one half of the curve is therefore 0.5.
Any fraction of total area represents relative frequency or probability. The
areas under half the curve are given from $z = 0$ to $z = 5$. Note that since the
curve is symmetrical, the area (always positive) from the mean of zero to a
negative value of z is the same as the area from zero to the same positive
value of z.

As an example, the area from $z = 0$ to $z = 1.44$ may be looked up
directly in the normal curve area table, and is 0.4251 (Figure 7.6).

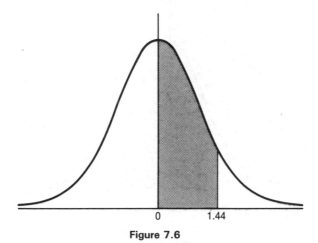

Figure 7.6

If the symmetrical area for $z = -1.44$ to $z = +1.44$ is required, the area
0.4251 is doubled to 0.8502. Other areas are obtained by adding or subtracting the areas from 0 to z, as demonstrated in Figure 7.7a, b, c and d.

Using the standard normal distribution we can obtain the proportion of
total frequency falling between specific values of the original data, after
first converting these into z-values.

Rather than starting from the z-values, we more commonly require to
look at a fixed percentage of total area under the normal curve, either area
in the tails of the distribution or central to it. The areas which will be
referred to subsequently and the corresponding z-values are shown in
Figure 7.8.

Where values are normally distributed, 68% lie between ± 1 standard
unit (or z-value), 95% lie between ± 1.96, 99% between ± 2.58 and 99.9%
between ± 3.3 standard units. These are very important relationships
which we shall use in discussing sampling in Chapters 8 and 10 to 12.

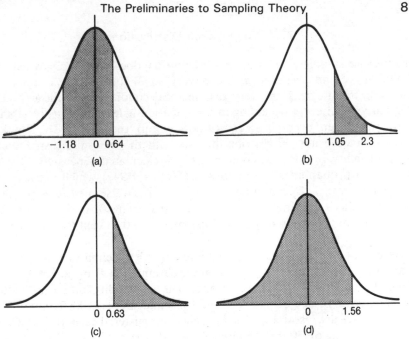

Figure 7.7

(a) The area from 0 to $z = -1.18$ is added to the area from 0 to $z = 0.64$ to obtain the area from $z = -1.18$ to $z = 0.64$;

(b) the area from 0 to $z = 1.05$ is subtracted from the area from 0 to $z = 2.3$ to obtain the area from $z = 1.05$ to $z = 2.3$;

(c) the area from 0 to $z = 0.63$ is subtracted from the area under half the curve (0.5) to obtain the area from $z = 0.63$ into the positive tail of the curve;

(d) the area from 0 to $z = 1.65$ is added to the area under half the curve (0.5) to obtain the area from the negative tail to $z = 1.65$.

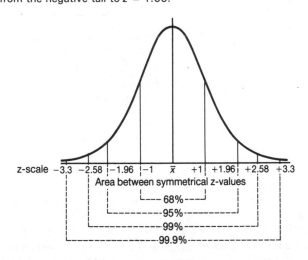

Figure 7.8

7.7 The Poisson Distribution

In studying samples, the normal distribution does not apply when the probability of an event occurring is very small indeed, for example in analysing the incidence of very rare medical conditions. If the expected frequency of an event occurring in a population is less than 5 (probability of the single event occurring × size of population), the Poisson Distribution is used, not the normal distribution. As with the binomial distribution, the probability of each outcome has to be calculated separately. Tables of Poisson probabilities are published (Molina, 1947) which provide the probability of 0, 1, 2 or more events occurring. To use the tables we need the probability of a single event occurring (suffering from a rare disease) and the size of the group or population exposed to the event (the number of people at risk).

Here is an example. Cancer registrations for leukaemia in England and Wales for persons under 15 years of age are running at approximately 4 per 100,000 population in that age group. The probability of an individual under 15 years of age being registered for leukaemia is 0.00004.

Suppose we are researching the incidence of registered cases of leukaemia in a population of 50,000 children under 15 years of age. On the basis of a probability of 0.00004 of any individual being so registered, we would expect 2 registered cases of leukaemia [0.00004 × 50,000 = 2] in this population. If we want to know the probability of getting more than 3 registered cases of leukaemia in a population of 50,000 children under 15 years of age, the Poisson Distribution would give the probabilities in Table 7.4.

Table 7.4 Probability of registered cases of leukaemia occurring

Number of cases	Probability	
0	0.1353	
1	0.2707	
2	0.2707	0.8571
3	0.1804	
4	0.0902	
5	0.0361	
6	0.0120	
7	0.0034	
8	0.0009	
9	0.0002	
10 or more	0.0001	
Total	1.0000	

The probability of getting 0 to 3 registered cases of leukaemia is 0.8571 (the sum of the separate probabilities of 0, 1, 2 or 3 cases occurring); the probability of getting 4 or more cases is 0.1429 [1 − 0.8571]. Thus the probability of getting 4 or more registered cases is one sixth of the probability of getting 0 to 3 cases [0.1429/0.8571 = 1/6]. What conclusions could be drawn depends on the context. Think of the arguments about the incidence of rare diseases and conditions, the cases of cancers and other conditions in the vicinity of nuclear power stations, chemical factories, waste tips, naturally occurring hazards etc., arguments which depend on calculations of this kind. Ultimately we face not certainty, but probability.

7.8   Summary

By the end of this chapter:

- you will understand the importance of the relationship between samples and populations;
- you will have a basic grasp of the meaning of random or probability sampling, and an understanding of the rules of probability;
- you have been introduced to the binomial distribution, the normal distribution, the standard normal distribution and the Poisson Distribution.

We shall build on your understanding of the normal distribution and the standard normal distribution in the chapters following.

Further Reading

For a light-hearted but sound introduction to probability.
Huff D (1973) *How to Take a Chance*. London: Penguin.

More demanding but worth trying:
Sprent P (1988) *Taking Risks: the Science of Uncertainty*. London: Penguin.

Other informal discussions of probability are to be found in:
Blalock H M (2nd edn 1979) *Social Statistics* Chapter 9. New York: McGraw-Hill.

Caulcott E (1973) *Significance Tests* Chapter 1 and 2. London: Routledge and Kegan Paul.

Hannagan T J (2nd edn 1988) *Mastering Statistics* Chapter 11. Basingstoke: Macmillan.

Moroney M J (1969) *Facts from Figures* Chapters 7, 8 and 9. London: Penguin.

A Little Practice

You have a bucket containing 1,000 marbles. Of these 600 are red, 300 are blue and 100 are white. The marbles are well mixed before each draw, and when drawing more than one marble you replace each marble before taking another.

1. You take a single marble out of the bucket. What is the probability of drawing (a) a red marble; (b) a blue marble; (c) either a blue marble or a white marble?

2. Now you draw two marbles. What is the probability of drawing (a) two blue marbles; (b) two white marbles; (c) a red marble and a white marble? (Remember to allow for the *two* outcomes, red followed by white and white followed by red.)

3. If you draw three marbles what is the probability (a) that all are white; (b) all are red; (c) one is white, one is red and one is blue? (Remember to allow for the several different colour orders in which you could draw the three marbles.)

8

Basic Ideas About Sampling: Sampling Theory

8.1 A Little Theory

Chapter 7 provided the underpinnings required for examining the relationship between random samples and the population from which they are drawn. We start with a little theory. Envisage that from a population a very large number of random samples of a fixed size are drawn, and that for each sample the mean is calculated. Commonsense (and Chapter 7) tells us that few of these many individual sample means will be exactly equal to the population mean. Commonsense also tells us that most of the sample means are likely to be fairly close to the mean of the population from which they come, with relatively few sample means greatly different from this population mean. The larger the sample size, the more closely we expect the sample means will be to the mean of the population. (Remember the effect of throwing 4 coins and 10 coins in Chapter 7.4; the theoretical pattern for the larger sample showed sample means clustered more closely round the population mean.)

Having obtained this large number of samples from a population and calculated the mean for each sample, we can put these values into a frequency distribution. This is called an 'experimental sampling distribution' because it is a distribution of sample values, obtained by experiment. The characteristics of this experimental sampling distribution will approximate closely to the characteristics of a theoretical sampling distribution. This latter is a normal distribution with mean equal to the population mean (μ), and standard deviation equal to the population standard deviation (σ) divided by the square root of sample size ($\sigma/\sqrt{n}$).* The theoretical sampling

---

* This relationship holds provided the population is distributed symmetrically. If the population distribution is skewed, the sampling distribution will also be skewed but to a very much lesser extent than the population itself (Croxton, Crowden and Klein, 1968, Chapter 24). For practical purposes the relationship between the experimental sampling distribution and the normal distribution holds.

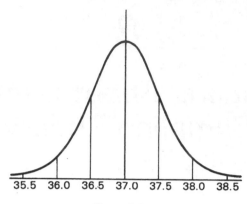

35.5   36.0   36.5   37.0   37.5   38.0   38.5

Figure 8.1

distribution is also a relative frequency or probability distribution because it demonstrates the frequency or probability with which particular sample means occur.

Suppose we drew a very large number of samples, size 100 (n), from a population with mean (μ) of 37 and standard deviation (σ) of 5, calculated the mean of each sample and constructed a frequency distribution with these sample means. We would expect this to approximate very closely to a normal distribution with a mean of 37 and a standard deviation of 0.5 ($\sigma\sqrt{n} = 5/\sqrt{100} = 0.5$). The theoretical distribution is shown in Figure 8.1.

In Chapter 7.6 we discussed the relationship between the area under the normal curve and both x- and z-values. Since the mean of the theoretical sampling distribution is 37 and its standard deviation is 0.5, we would expect 95% of all the sample means to lie between 37 ± 1.96 × 0.5, that is, between 37 ± 0.98, or 36.02 and 37.98. Similarly we would expect 99% of the sample means to lie between 37 ± 2.58 × 0.5, or 35.71 and 38.29, and 99.9% to lie between 37 ± 3.3 × 0.5, or 35.35 and 38.65.

Expressed in general algebraic terms expectation is that:

95%   of sample means lie between $\mu \pm 1.96 \times \sigma/\sqrt{n}$
99%   of sample means lie between $\mu \pm 2.58 \times \sigma/\sqrt{n}$
99.9% of sample means lie between $\mu \pm 3.3 \times \sigma/\sqrt{n}$.

The same principles hold for percentages. Although proportion/percentages follow the binomial distribution (Chapter 7.4 and 7.5), the normal distribution is used as an approximation for the binomial distribution. The binomial distribution for percentages has a mean percentage equal to $\theta\%$ (pronounced theta), the population percentage, and a standard deviation of $\sqrt{\theta\%(100 - \theta)\%/n}$. Exactly the same general statements can be made about the distributions of sample percentages as about the distribution of sample means:

95% of sample percentages lie between $\theta\% \pm 1.96 \times \sqrt{\dfrac{\theta\%(100 - \theta)\%}{n}}$

99% of sample percentages lie between $\theta\% \pm 2.58 \times \sqrt{\dfrac{\theta\%(100 - \theta)\%}{n}}$

99.9% of sample percentages lie between $\theta\% \pm 3.3 \times \sqrt{\dfrac{\theta\%(100 - \theta)\%}{n}}$

Let us pursue these points with examples.

8.2 A Little Practice—Means

We need a convenient population from which to derive samples, and will use hospital dental staff (England) by age at 30 September 1987.* This population consist of 1,235 dentists; their age distribution is set in out in Table 8.1 and the histogram in Figure 8.2. Note that the mean age of this population of dentists is 39.34 years, and the standard deviation is 12.47 years. These measures have been calculated from the original ages, not from the grouped data.[†]

Table 8.1   Age of hospital dental staff 1987

Age in years	Number of dentists
20 and under 25	157
25 and under 30	241
30 and under 35	123
35 and under 40	120
40 and under 45	160
45 and under 50	129
50 and under 55	109
55 and under 60	111
60 and under 65	77
65 and under 70	7
70 and under 75	1
All ages	1,235

---

* This is the same group of dentists as shown in Table 5.3. Whereas Table 5.3 is published data, Table 8.1 is derived from the original (unpublished) data.

[†] It is for this reason that these measures differ from those we calculated from the grouped data in Chapters 5 and 6.

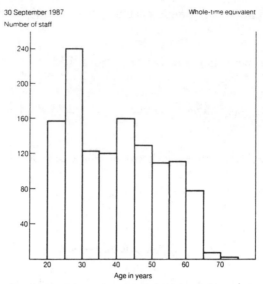

Figure 8.2 Age of hospital dental staff, England

Using a computer program, random samples were generated from this data, together with the mean of each sample. To make a useful comparison, sample sizes of 50 dentists, and sample sizes of 100 dentists were drawn. For each sample size, two separate groups of 100 random samples were drawn. For each group of 100 samples, mean and standard deviation were calculated, and also the mean and standard deviation of the combined groups of 200 of each sample size. These are shown in Table 8.2 together with the mean (μ) and standard deviation ($\sigma/\sqrt{n}$) of the theoretical sampling distributions.

Table 8.2 Samples of hospital dental staff: age in years at 30.9.87

	Mean	Standard deviation
Sample size 50		
A 100 samples	39.31	1.64
B 100 samples	39.41	1.93
A + B 200 samples	39.36	1.80
Sampling distribution	39.34	1.76
Sample size 100		
C 100 samples	39.30	1.22
D 100 samples	39.40	1.26
C + D 200 samples	39.35	1.24
Sampling distribution	39.34	1.25

The means of all the sampling distributions are reasonably close to the mean of the theoretical sampling distributions, as are the standard deviations of the sampling distributions to the standard deviations of the theoretical sampling distributions. Generally the figures are closer for the combined groups of 200 samples than for the separate groups of 100 samples, emphasising the importance of sampling distributions being based on *large* numbers of samples.

Histograms for the combined samples are shown in Figure 8.3, demonstrating the bell shape of the experimental sampling distributions, centred approximately on the population mean. Note the wider dispersion of the distribution of samples size 50 compared with samples size 100.

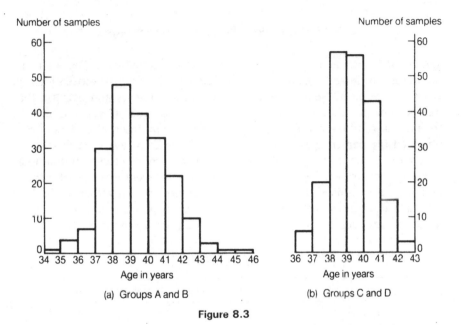

(a) Groups A and B   (b) Groups C and D

Figure 8.3

Table 8.3 Sample means: observed and expected patterns

Range of values	Age range in years	No. of samples outside range	
		Observed	Expected
A + B (200 samples, size 50)			
95% range $\mu \pm 1.96\ \sigma/\sqrt{n}$	35.89 to 42.80	11	10
99% range $\mu \pm 2.58\ \sigma/\sqrt{n}$	34.79 to 43.89	3	2
C + D (200 samples, size 100)			
95% range $\mu \pm 1.96\ \sigma/\sqrt{n}$	36.90 to 41.79	8	10
99% range $\mu \pm 2.58\ \sigma/\sqrt{n}$	36.12 to 42.56	1	2

Now to relate theory and practice by considering the number of sample means which fall outside the ranges of value discussed in section 1 above, and the number of samples expected so to fall. Comparison is clearer if we look at the small numbers of samples outside these ranges, rather than the very much larger numbers within the ranges, as shown in Table 8.3.

These results are quite close. In two instances the observed samples outside the range exceed the theoretical number expected; in the other two outcomes the observed samples are fewer than the theoretical number expected. A reasonable degree of coincidence, especially as the total number of samples in each case (200) is quite small. A much larger number of samples would provide closer agreement between theory and practice.

8.3 A Little More Practice—Percentages

The same experiments can be repeated with percentages. Consider the population of hospital dental staff divided into two groups; those under 40 years of age on 30 September 1987, and those 40 years and over on that date. Of the population of dentists, 51.90% were under 40 years of age. As for means, random samples were generated by computer from which were obtained the percentage of dentists under 40 years of age in each sample. Two groups each of 100 samples size 50 and two groups each of 100 samples size 100 were drawn. Table 8.4 shows the mean percentages in each group, and in the combined groups for each sample size, together with their standard deviations. For comparison, the mean percentage and standard deviation for each of the theoretical sampling distributions is also shown.

Table 8.4 Samples of hospital dental staff: percentages under 40 years of age at 30.9.87

	Mean percentage	Standard deviation
Sample size 50		
E 100 samples	52.94	7.05
F 100 samples	51.32	7.73
E + F 200 samples	52.13	7.42
Sampling distribution	51.90	7.07
Sample size 100		
G 100 samples	51.90	4.84
H 100 samples	51.72	5.48
G + H 200 samples	51.81	5.15
Sampling distribution	51.90	5.00

As for the sample means, Figure 8.4 shows the histograms for the combined distributions of percentages from samples of different size. This again

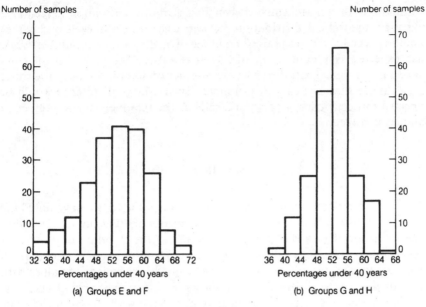

Figure 8.4

demonstrates the noticeably wider spread of the distribution derived from the smaller samples. Both distributions are centred approximately on the population percentage.

We again look at the relationship between the empirical distribution of sample percentages against their theoretical distribution.

Table 8.5 Sample percentages: observed and expected patterns

Range of values	Percentage range	No. of samples outside range	
		Observed	Expected
E + F (200 samples, size 50)			
95% range $\theta\% \pm 1.96 \times \sqrt{\dfrac{\theta\%(100 - \theta)\%}{n}}$	38.051 to 65.749	12	10
99% range $\theta\% \pm 2.58 \times \sqrt{\dfrac{\theta\%(100 - \theta)\%}{n}}$	33.670 to 70.130	1	2
G + H (200 samples, size 100)			
95% range $\theta\% \pm 1.96 \times \sqrt{\dfrac{\theta\%(100 - \theta)\%}{n}}$	42.107 to 61.693	14	10
99% range $\theta\% \pm 2.58 \times \sqrt{\dfrac{\theta\%(100 - \theta)\%}{n}}$	39.010 to 64.790	0	2

Looking at the relationship between the distribution of sample percentages and their theoretical distribution, in two cases the observed number of samples exceed the expected; in the other two, the observed number is less than expected. We note in one of these cases (the 95% range for the combined samples size 100), the observed number of samples outside the range is four more than the expected number. Such a large difference would be expected to occur occasionally, and reflects the relatively small number of samples involved.

8.4   A Little of Both

In relating theory and practice in sections 2 and 3 above, we have noted the closeness of the relationship between the means of the sampling distributions (whether of means or percentages), and of the standard deviations of these sample statistics, to the theoretically expected measures. Comparison of the actual number of sample measures outside the ranges of values with the numbers theoretically expected shows a reasonable coincidence. The histograms demonstrate an approximate bell shape with a concentration of the sampling distributions round the population means; the distributions of samples size 100 clearly show a narrower spread than the distributions of samples size 50. Theory and the empirical evidence run together.

We now have the basis for establishing what conclusions can be drawn about a population from the information contained in a single sample. Before developing this we need to explore matters pertaining to sampling and research design in Chapter 9.

8.5   Summary

From this chapter:

- you have learnt about the relationship between experimental sampling distributions (means and percentages) and the characteristics of the population from which the samples are drawn;
- you understand the important role of the normal distribution in this relationship;
- in looking at sampling distributions, you are aware that:

1. the mean of the sampling distribution will be close to the population mean. This applies also to the mean percentage of a sampling distribution and the population percentage;
2. the dispersion in the sampling distribution (standard deviation) reflects the dispersion in the population;

3. the larger the size of the samples drawn, the smaller the dispersion in the sampling distribution. The effect is a reduction by the square root of sample size;
4. sampling distributions are relative frequency or probability distributions; they reflect the relative frequency or probability with which specific values occur.

Further Reading

Sample and population and sampling distributions are discussed in:

Caulcott E (1973) *Significance Tests* Chapter 3. London: Routledge and Kegan Paul.
Freund J E and Williams F J (1970 2nd edn) *Modern Business Statistics* Chapter 8. Bath: Pitman.
Hoel P G and Jessen R J (1977 2nd edn) *Basic Statistics for Business and Economics* Chapter 6. New York: Wiley.
Reichmann W J *Use and Abuse of Statistics* (1964) Chapter 15. London: Penguin.

A Little Practice

Try these with the aid of some friends.

1. Toss four coins for heads. Get at least 100 results, more if possible. Turn your results into a percentage distribution of number of heads and compare with the theoretical distribution from Table 7.2. The theoretical percentages are given by multiplying the last column (probability) by 100. Then calculate (a) the mean *number* of heads and (b) the standard deviation for your results and compare with the theoretical mean and standard deviation given with the answers.

2. Repeat 1 above with 10 coins, and compare your distribution with Table 7.3. Calculate the mean and standard deviation for the number of heads from your results.

9

Sampling and Research Designs

9.1 Problems of Populations

The discussions in Chapters 7 and 8 are based on the simple random sample drawn from a known population. In an ideal world we can identify every unit in the population, and for sampling purposes, can attribute to each unit a known non-zero probability of selection, often an equal probability of selection. The sample results relate to this known population.

Identifying the population in this way is not always possible. Much research in the nursing/medical field is about comparisons between groups of individuals, people in specific circumstances, patients suffering from a particular condition. Such groups are not selected randomly from the population of all who suffer from a particular condition. If patients are from one hospital only, or from one community health area only, they are drawn from a limited population—those in the particular hospital or community health area. They represent patients diagnosed and recorded, not all those suffering from the particular condition, and may well consist of patients whose condition is more severe, more advanced. Because patients are 'accessible' for research does not necessarily mean that research will provide information of application outside the specific group on which the research is conducted.

Early research on smoking and lung cancer used males who were suffering from lung cancer and compared these with other groups; 'healthy men of the same age groups', or male patients suffering from other forms of cancer, or being treated for other conditions. What was established was that smoking was more common amongst lung cancer patients. These small-scale research studies could only provide a pointer; both the lung cancer patients and other patients were self-selected groups, not random samples drawn from defined populations. Further research was necessary, which had to be more rigorously designed in order that conclusions could be drawn from the research results (Doll and Hill, 1950).

There are two questions to consider. Firstly, if we draw conclusions about the patients in this hospital or that community health area, does this justify an extension of the conclusions to a wider area, a more general population? If looking at samples drawn from two populations, and seeking to compare sample results, we can only do so in terms of the characteristics of the populations from which the samples are drawn. The question of the population(s) being sampled requires careful thought and adequate definition.

Secondly, within the limitations of the population(s) being sampled, can we look upon these samples as random samples? Are samples selected randomly from the total group in the single hospital or the community health area? There may have been a certain element of fortuitousness in the individuals selected—for example, patients registered after a particular date. If so, can we treat these as random samples of all patients currently registering for treatment of this condition? In order to do so, we would need to be reasonably confident that the patients from whom the samples were selected were not from some special or different group which would lead to bias in the research results.

9.2   The Sampling Frame

Consider a research study based on all patients who have registered for treatment for a specific condition at a group of hospitals during a defined time-period. The first step is to identify each unit within this population.

The means of so doing is called the sampling frame. This could be the hospital record number for each patient. Alternatively, each patient when registering could be given a number in sequence and this special list used as a sampling frame. A wider population within the community could be based on lists of NHS patients registered with general medical practitioners. But patients move away or die and records are not updated; general medical practitioners' lists will not include all the residents in an area. All lists have deficiencies which must be taken into account when designing research and drawing research conclusions.

A sampling frame may be more elaborate than a single list. A study covering several hospitals could be based on a separate list for each hospital, which would have advantages at the point of sample selection. The same principles would apply to the drawing up of each separate list.

The sampling frame is a means of identifying all units of a population in a way in which the identification can be used as a basis for sample selection. We need to be aware who is included and who is excluded from the sampling frame. Omissions are important, and can have a profound effect on research conclusions.

9.3   Sample Selection

Before selecting the sample, we will have defined the population, either through a sampling frame, or within a specific framework, as by letting it consist of patients registered after a particular date. Using this sampling frame, we select a random sample from the research population.

If the sampling frame is a list of patients, selection from this list is made in such a way that we are reasonably confident the sample selected is a random sample. If it is a list of patients by hospital numbers (which need not be in continuous sequence), or a specially drawn list of sequential numbers, we can use tables of random numbers to make a random selection (Rand Corporation, 1966).* In the first case when numbers not on the list were drawn these would be ignored. For both list types, we would select patients through random numbers until the target sample size was achieved.

Another way of dealing with a list of patients is to select sample patients at regular intervals through the list. This is known as an interval sample, and is satisfactory in most circumstances provided there is no periodicity in the list itself, that is, the names in the list can be looked upon as being in random order. The sampling interval (the gap between patients selected from the list) would be N/n where N is the size of the population (number of names on the list) and n is the target sample size. See section 5 following for an example of how this operates.

An alternative situation is when research is based on an ongoing population, for example new patients first registering after a given date. Provided that from knowledge of previous patients we can be fairly certain that current patients register in a haphazard fashion, not clustering by relevant characteristics, a sample drawn from newly registered patients will be unbiased and can be treated as a random sample.

9.4 Experimental Design

Research using experimental design is common in the health field. Two or more groups are studied on a before and after basis. The characteristic of interest is measured in each group before treatment, the different treatments are applied, and the outcomes measured after treatment.

The crucial point is that the measurable change following treatment should be attributable only to the treatment and due neither to differences between the initial sample groups nor to additional factors not allowed for in the study. We need to be sure that no extraneous influences have crept in. Only the treatment should be a possible 'cause' of different outcomes.

Such a research design requires random samples. How can we ensure this? How can we minimise the risk that at the commencement of the research, one group is different from the other in some material way?

---

* Many statistics textbooks include sample pages of random numbers which could be used for a small scale research study.

Suppose that age at the time of registering when suffering from a particular condition is important; possibly the young recover more quickly. If there were a disproportionate number of young people in one group receiving a new treatment that might account for the results of the study suggesting the new treatment is more effective than the old treatment. Had the groups been similar as regards age distribution, the outcome of the study might have been quite different.

We have to solve such problems. Starting with the total group of patients available to the study (the population), we may be able to draw two random samples by means of a table of random numbers, and to allocate these to the two methods of treatment. Differences between the samples in relevant characteristics would then be subject only to sampling error (see Chapters 10 to 14).

If patients are included in the research study on an ongoing basis as they first register after a particular date, we could allocate them in turn to the two groups. That would be satisfactory provided the order of registering was virtually random.* Alternatively, to avoid the possibility of considerable variation between the groups, we could match patients either:

1. by matching pairs of patients on relevant variables, and then randomly assigning each of a pair to one of the two groups; or

2. by ensuring similar frequency distributions of relevant variables in each group.

Either approach improves the efficiency of the research design, provided a random method is used to allocate patients to each group.

What might be relevant variables? These are determined by the nature of the study itself, but might include sex, age, socio-economic characteristics, length of time suffering from the condition, behaviour related to the condition. The aim is to include all variables which might be relevant to the subject of the study, and for which information is available.

The first method involves matching individuals (which can be difficult); the second aims at ensuring that the two samples contain approximately the same proportions by sex, age category, severity of condition and so on. By these means, we seek to minimise the risk of starting the study with samples which are not comparable.

We must also ensure that errors do not creep in during the course of the research and distort the results. This is a different problem, related to ongoing research, not one to be dealt with here, but which is covered in standard textbooks on research methods.

---

* Even if there were some clustering, for example, men tending to register at the beginning of the week and women at the end, the allocation alternately to the two groups would ensure equal distribution to the groups.

9.5 Experimental Design—An Example

These points can be examined through an example. We are researching hospital patients with a particular skin condition and wish to base the research on the first 80 new patients registering after a given date. Patients are to be divided into two groups, one to receive a new treatment (experimental group), the other to receive the old treatment (control group). For the research to be valid, these patients need to be similar to other patients with this skin condition who register at the hospital. Suppose the hospital gets approximately 300 new patients registering each year for treatment of the skin condition. The 80 research patients would register in a period of approximately three months from the starting date. If the research had started at a different time of year, would this make any difference? Provided all previous evidence was that there was no material difference between patients and outcomes whatever the time of year at which they registered, and that their registration was an unbiased event, the first 80 patients registering after a particular date would be a suitable sample. But what if the skin condition is affected by the season of the year, and the serious cases occur in August and September? This could have a profound effect. If the study period excluded August and September, we would select disproportionately few of the most serious cases; if it included August and September, the research would be heavily weighted with serious cases. So what can be done?

One solution would be to extend the research period to a full 12 months to get a complete range of seasonal effects. This would have two disadvantages. Firstly, that there would be a lapse of 12 months (not just over 3 months) between the selection of the first sample patient and the last sample patient. This would add 9 months to the research project, which could pose problems. Secondly, a year's patients would number approximately 300. If the study is to be limited to 80 patients, and resources are not available to study 300 patients, we need a means of reducing 300 patients to 80. This can be by a form of random selection. We will register all new patients and take, not every patient, but patients at intervals through the list, using a sampling interval calculated as:

$$\frac{\text{expected number of patients in 12 months}}{\text{required sample size}} = \frac{300}{80} = 3.75.^*$$

---

* This is a general principle. The required sampling interval always equals:

$$\frac{\text{(anticipated) population size}}{\text{target sample size}}.$$

In order to sample through the list of patients, we need a random number start,* being a number between 1 and 3 (the 3 being the whole number part of the sampling interval). The first sample patient is the one on the list coinciding with the random number start. The second sample patient is obtained by adding the sampling interval to the random number start, the third by adding the sampling interval again.[†] This is done cumulatively, and taken through the list of new patients will provide a sample of the size we want. The method provides unbiased selection, with each new patient registering having an equal probability of selection. Further, there is commonly a degree of randomness in the registration of patients which also contributes to the randomness of the process.

Alternatively, we could incorporate stratification techniques in the selection of 80 patients newly registered with the skin condition. With careful definition of the categories and making use of past records, we could estimate the proportions of patients who had suffered mildly, moderately and severely from the skin condition. Either each group could be studied separately, or samples drawn which had the same proportions of mild, moderate and severe cases as had occurred in the past. Suppose the proportions were 45% mild, 35% moderate and 20% severe. A sample of 80 should contain 36 mild cases (45% of 80), 28 moderate cases (35% of 80) and 16 severe cases (20% of 80).

As new patients registered after the study had started, we would collect information about them, assess the severity of the condition and decide into which category each patient fell. The study would consist of the first 36 mild cases, the first 28 moderate cases and the first 16 severe cases registered. In this way the overall pattern of mild, moderate and severe cases would be reflected in the sample.

---

* We can obtain this using a table of random numbers. Alternatively, a quick method of selecting a single random number is to use a large telephone directory which contains several hundred pages, all numbered. Flick the pages through, shut your eyes, open the book at random. Use the *tens* digit from the page number on the open page as a random number. If it is not within the range required, here between 1 and 3, repeat until it is.

[†] Suppose the random number start is 2. This is what happens.

Sample patient selected		Order of registration
First	2	2nd patient
Second	2 + 3.75 = 5.75	5th patient
Third	5.75 + 3.75 = 9.5	9th patient
Fourth	9.5 + 3.75 = 13.25	13th patient
Fifth	13.25 + 3.75 = 17	17th patient
Sixth	17 + 3.75 = 20.75	20th patient
Seventh	20.75 + 3.75 = 24.5	24th patient
Eighth	24.5 + 3.75 = 28.25	28th patient
Ninth	28.25 + 3.75 = 32	32nd patient
Tenth	32 + 3.75 = 35.75	35th patient
Eleventh	35.75 + 3.75 = 39.5	39th patient
And so on.		

Dividing the patients into two groups, an experimental group and a control group, we would use a random method to allocate individual mild, moderate and severe cases to the two groups, or use a matching technique described in section 4 above.

This is an example of the general principle of stratification which can be used to improve the quality of a sample. The stratification factor, here the severity of the condition, must be relevant to the research in question. In theory it is possible to use more than one stratification factor, but more than one adds greatly to the complication of sample design and may not produce a corresponding benefit.*

9.6 Replication

If research results are not conclusive, the means of resolving this is to take further samples, replicating the study, aggregating results and thereby increasing overall sample size. Initial research design should take account of this requirement.

Take the example of patients suffering from a particular skin condition (divided into three categories of mild, moderate and severe cases). Using the method of sampling throughout a twelve month period, we can replicate the sample by extending it over another twelve months. The second sample need not be of identical size. If other than 80 cases were required in the second year a revised sampling interval would be used.

Had we used a stratification technique, dividing newly registered cases into mild, moderate and severe cases, further patients would be selected in each category to a new target sample size. This again would be divided pro rata to the distribution of 45% mild cases, 35% moderate cases and 20% severe cases.

9.7 Measurement

Defining what is to be measured is of profound importance. Measurement sounds straightforward but can involve difficulties of definition and the problem of avoiding bias. Clear and meaningful criteria are required for measurement, criteria which can be operated in an independent, systematic and unbiased way. If deciding whether patients are suffering moderately, mildly or severely, we require an agreed method of achieving a decision on the category to which to allocate each patient. If seeking to decide whether

---

*If adding age as a second stratification factor, say in three categories, we would have [3 × 3 = 9] groups into which to allocate the original sample.

patients in a study have reached a particular level of improvement in the condition from which they are suffering, that level must be defined in terms of agreed and operable criteria before the study starts. The criteria decided upon should produce the same outcomes whoever is operating them; the measurement technique must be reliable. If an element of subjective assessment enters in, more than one 'assessor' may be necessary and a system developed for achieving a final decision. We must be aware of what we are doing, not have expectations regarding patients' progress, and be able to reach a reliable and consistent assessment which operates equally in regard to all patients.

9.8 A Final Point

This chapter directs our thoughts to issues in research, and deals briefly with some of the more important aspects linking sampling and research designs. It is not a substitute for the greater detail in texts dealing with research methodology. Looking at these issues provides a necessary background to the following five chapters which are concerned with the conclusions which can be drawn from research studies based on random samples.

For those seriously concerned either in designing research or in assessing the quality of the results of existing research, further reading is suggested below.

9.9 Summary

- You have examined some basic points about samples and research design;
- you know about the need to define the population under study and the issues involved in selecting an unbiased sample;
- you have been introduced to the sampling frame, and the way in which a sample can be selected from it;
- you are aware of the place of experimental designs in research, particularly important in the health field, and how these may be constituted;
- you appreciate the need to structure designs so that the study can be replicated.

Finally, you will always remember the need to define, in practical and relevant terms, that which is to be measured.

Further Reading

Bulmer M (1984) *Sociological Research Methods: An Introduction.* London: Macmillan.

Couchman C and Dawson J (1990) *Nursing and Health Care Research.* London: Scutari.

Hakim C (1987) *Research Design.* London: Allen and Unwin.

Hill A B (1962) *Statistical Methods in Clinical and Preventive Medicine.* Edinburgh: Livingstone. These collected papers are well worth attention. See particularly Chapters 1, 10, 15 and 16.

Moser C and Kalton G (1971 2nd edn) *Survey Methods in Social Investigation* Chapters 5–7 and 9. London: Heinemann.

Ogier M E (1989) *Reading Research.* London: Scutari.

Oppenheim A N (1966) *Questionnaire Design and Attitude Measurement.* London: Heinemann.

Polgar S and Thomas S A (1988) *Introduction to Research in the Health Sciences* Chapters 1–3. Melbourne: Churchill Livingstone.

Interlude — Data and Levels of Measurement

Before starting on the following important chapters on statistical inference and Part IV on analysis, we need to reflect on data, on the levels of measurement we discussed in Chapter 2.3, the appropriateness of the methods and tests of Chapters 10 to 14, and the analytical techniques of Chapters 15 and 16.

Where we are dealing with means which are computed measures, the underlying level of measurement is interval. Our data must be parametric. This applies to the data used for the estimation of population means of Chapter 10.1 to 10.6, the tests covering sample and population means of Chapter 11.1 to 11.4, the differences between two or more sample means of Chapter 12.1 and 12.2 and Chapter 14. There should be no difficulty here in recognising the appropriateness of techniques in relation to the data.

When we are dealing with percentages we are commonly dealing with non-parametric data, that is nominal or ordinal levels of measurement. Percentages are based on a simple head counting exercise; who possesses a particular characteristic. If we are dealing with a simple dichotomy—possession of the characteristic or not—we are dealing strictly with a nominal level of measurement. This is a very simple form of data and many situations can be so structured. 'Was the patient's recovery speedy or slow?' can be restructured as 'Was the patient discharged not later than the fifth day after the operation?'. The two questions are not the same, but the second provides a straightforward objective criterion by which patients can be placed in one of two categories. The objective criterion requires a logically sound basis which can be altered if it appears to make an insufficiently clear distinction between speedy and less speedy recovery. This simple nominal dichotomy is the basis for the estimation of population percentages of Chapter 10.7, tests covering population and sample percentages of Chapter 11.5 and tests for differences between two sample percentages of Chapter 12.3.

If we are concerned with data subdivided into more than two categories, the level of measurement may be nominal or ordinal. For example, whether patients experience mild, moderate or severe pain, shows a clear ordering of the data. The chi-square test of Chapter 13 handles the proportionate (equivalent to percentage) distribution of data across a number of subgroups, and properly handles both nominal and ordinal data. This test can also be used for interval data, but is of particular importance for its ability to accommodate non-parametric data. It is a widely used and flexible test which can handle virtually any data.

The methods of analysis described in Chapters 15 and 16 formally require parametric, that is interval data, such as for individual patients, the number of days of treatment for a condition to achieve a specific degree of improvement. The exception to this is the rank correlation coefficient of Chapter 16.6 which will handle ordinal data as well as interval data, and for this reason is particular useful.

When seeking to apply suitable methods and tests for analysing and interpreting data, especially research data, think carefully not only about the data itself, but about how you can organise it. Rethinking the data and the situation into a form suitable for testing or analysis is a useful starting point. Be aware of the level of measurement of your data and how this relates to the methods to be used.

The tests and techniques of the remainder of this book are 'robust' in that they enable firm conclusions to be drawn. For non-parametric data there are additional tests which can be used, and suitable references are given. Great caution is needed in using and interpreting these weaker tests as they often lead to somewhat indeterminate conclusions. What they may do is to provide guidance for further research, the results of which can be made the subject of the more robust tests described here.

Before starting on any tests of research data, the data itself needs careful inspection (see Chapter 4). This may well provide as much information and guidance as a weak non-parametric test.

10

Estimation: Conclusions From the Single Sample

10.1 Estimating the Population Mean—95% Confidence Limits

In the last three chapters we have explored ideas about probability and sampling distributions, and about the relationship between sampling and research design. The discussions in Chapters 7 and 8 were of situations involving many samples drawn from a known population. The research aspects of Chapter 9 were concerned with problems of drawing a sample from a population so that from that sample valid conclusions could be reached about the population. Given that the sample is suitably drawn and can be looked upon as a random sample, what can be inferred from it?

If we draw many samples, size 100, from the population of 1,235 hospital dentists (Chapter 8) we know that 95% of the samples will have means which lie within the range of $[\mu \pm 1.96 \times \sigma/\sqrt{n}]$ or $[39.34 \pm (1.96 \times 1.247)]$ years, that is, between 36.90 years and 41.79 years. If we draw a single sample, its mean will have a probability of 0.95 (95%) of falling within these limits. Suppose we know nothing about the population, but have a single sample of 100 hospital dentists, and the sample has a mean age of 38.79 years with standard deviation 12.44 years. This could have come from a number of different populations, different in terms of their means. How can we establish something about the 'true' population mean? Starting with the sample mean as the 'best estimate' of the population mean we can obtain a range of values within which we would expect the 'true' population mean to lie. Additionally we require an estimate of the standard deviation of the population. For this purpose, we use the sample standard deviation (s) as 'best estimate' of the population standard deviation, and obtain an estimate $s/\sqrt{n}$ for the standard deviation of the sampling distribution.

From the single sample we have a mean ($\bar{x}$) of 38.79 years, used as an estimate of the population mean (μ), and a standard deviation (s) of 12.44 years from which is derived the estimate of $\sigma/\sqrt{n}$ as $12.44/\sqrt{100}$ or 1.244 years.

The argument about the relationship between sample and population means can be turned round. Recollecting that sampling distributions are relative frequency or probability distributions, we can say that there is a probability of 0.95 (95%) that the sample comes from a population whose mean lies between $[\bar{x} \pm 1.96 \times s/\sqrt{n}]$ or $[38.79 \pm (1.96 \times 1.244)]$ years, that is between 36.35 and 41.23 years. Note that the mean of the population, 39.34 years does lie between these values.* This range is called the 95% confidence limits, because we are (on account of the statistical method used) 95% confident that the population mean lies within it.

10.2 The Standard Error

Pause for a moment to consider the measure $\sigma/\sqrt{n}$ for which the 'best estimate' is $s/\sqrt{n}$. It is the standard deviation of the sampling distribution and is a measure of the possible error involved in using the sample mean as the 'best estimate' of the population mean. Further it is the theoretical measure of difference between the (known) sample mean, and the (unknown) population mean. This measure of error is known as the standard error, here the standard error of the mean.

Standard errors are the standard deviations of sampling distributions. All sample statistics have a calculable standard error, and the term 'standard error' is generic. We refer to specific standard errors as appropriate, for example, the standard error of the mean, the standard error of the percentage. As a shorthand, we abbreviate 'standard error' to 'se', adding an appropriate subscript. The standard error of the mean is '$se_{\bar{x}}$'. In all future discussions the term 'standard error' will be used when referring to the standard deviation of a sampling distribution.

10.3 Estimating the Population Mean — More Confidence Limits

The probability that the population mean lies within a given range of values can be increased, but at the expense of widening this range. Following discussions in Chapter 8, we can say that there is a probability of 0.99 (99%) that the population mean lies within the range $[\bar{x} \pm 2.58 \times se_{\bar{x}}]$ or $[38.79 \pm (2.58 \times 1.244)]$ years, that is, between 35.58 years and 42.00 years. These are the 99% confidence limits. The probability of being right is higher (0.99 compared with 0.95), but the answer is less precise—a wider range of values. Similarly 99.9% confidence limits are $[\bar{x} \pm 3.3 \times se_{\bar{x}}]$,

---

*Whilst there is a 95% probability of being right when saying the population mean lies within this range, there is a 5% probability of being wrong, a 5% probability that the population mean lies below 36.35 years or above 41.23 years.

[38.79 ± (3.3 × 1.244]) years, or 34.68 to 42.90 years. Greater confidence in the results is at the price of even less precision. The relationships are shown in Figure 10.1.

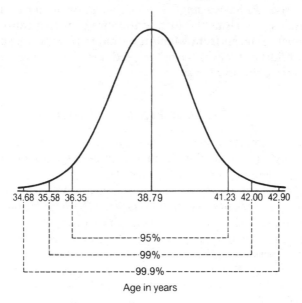

Age in years

Figure 10.1 Age in years of hospital dental staff 1987: confidence limits

Why use 95%, 99% and 99.9% confidence limits? Because on the whole these 'work'. Data in samples based on health or social measures tend to be fairly variable, and 95% confidence limits are commonly used. For greater confidence but with less precision we could select 99% confidence limits, but it is most unlikely we would need to consider the 99.9% confidence limits. These are more appropriate for scientific and engineering work where a high degree of accuracy is common. In some fields, notably business and commerce, the narrower 90% confidence limits may be used.*

We could construct any other confidence limits required, making use of the normal curve properties to do so. But the use of 95%, 99% and 99.9% confidence limits is well established, and widely accepted.

All estimates based on samples are subject to sampling error, the error attributable to the sampling process, of which the standard error is a measure. Research results based on samples (for example, mean number of occupied beds, mean length of stay as an in-patient, mean lapse of time to

---

* The 90% confidence limits would be obtained from

$$\bar{x} \pm 1.65 \times se_{\bar{x}}.$$

Major official surveys, such as the Family Expenditure Survey or the NES quote standard errors against their estimates from which any desired confidence limits can be derived.

specific improvement) cannot properly be interpreted without reference to the standard error. Confidence limits are a convenient way of expressing this error.

To summarise: we have a single sample, we know its mean, its standard deviation and its size. Using this information we construct confidence limits for the population mean from which the sample is drawn. The method of obtaining confidence limits is set out in section 5, but before pursuing this, there is another point to discuss.

10.4　The Small Population Correction

This is a good moment to dismiss a fallacy and to introduce a refinement.

The accuracy of information from a sample depends on the absolute sample size—how many units in the sample. The square root of absolute sample size *always* appears in the denominator of the expression for a standard error. It does not matter how large is the population from which a sample is drawn. That is just as well, since often we are dealing with populations either of unknown size or of infinite size (such as ongoing populations of persons suffering from particular conditions).

The fallacy to be dismissed is that the *percentage* of the population sampled matters. It is largely irrelevant. A small percentage sample drawn from a large population may be numerically larger than a large sample from a small population. For example, 5% of a population of 40,000 is 2,000; that will produce a more accurate result (because it will generate a smaller standard error) than a 10% sample from a population of 5,000, which is 500. The size of the population from which a sample is drawn is seldom of serious interest.

Having said that, we should note a correction for use when the population is small in relation to a sample. It is not worth considering unless a sample is at least 5% of the population, and it is only when the sample is around 10% of the population that the correction makes a material difference.

The formula for the small population correction is:

$$\sqrt{\frac{N - n}{N - 1}}$$

where N is the size of the population and n is the size of the sample. The standard error is multiplied by this correction (which must be less than 1), so the effect is to reduce the standard error.

Consider the effect on a sample drawn from the population of hospital dentists. For a sample size 100, the small population correction would be:

$$\sqrt{\frac{1,235 - 100}{1,235 - 1}} = \sqrt{\frac{1,135}{1,234}} = \sqrt{0.9198} = 0.959.$$

Multiplying the standard error by this correction:

$$se_{\bar{x}} = 1.244 \times 0.959 = 1.193.$$

Using this correction, the 95% confidence limits for the population from which the single sample is drawn would be 36.45 to 41.13 years. The 99% confidence limits would be 35.71 to 41.87 years and the 99.9% confidence limits 34.85 to 42.73 years.

The correction, at 0.959, reduces the standard error and the width of the confidence limits by 4.1% (100% − 95.9%). Not a very great improvement, which is hardly surprising because the sample size, 100, is 8% of the population. Had sample size been 200, and 16% of the population, the correction would be 0.916. The percentage reduction in standard error and confidence limits would have been approximately 8.4%.

There are not many occasions when we can gain materially by using the small population correction. A convenient rule of thumb is to use it if the sample is at least 5% of the population.* Ignoring the correction is not a positive error. We should know it exists, and remember to use it if the population is noticeably small in relation to sample size.

10.5   An Example

When establishing confidence limits, start by calculating the standard error first (adjusted by the small population correction if this is appropriate), and then obtain the confidence limits. Suppose we require confidence limits for the mean length of stay in hospital of dermatology patients. We have information on 174 patients whose mean length of stay was 19.2 days, with standard deviation 4.1 days. On the basis that this is a simple random sample we proceed as follows.

1. Start by setting out the information in terms of algebraic notation:

$$\bar{x} = 19.2 \text{ days} \qquad \text{(sample mean)}$$
$$s = 4.1 \text{ days} \qquad \text{(sample standard deviation)}$$
$$n = 174 \text{ patients} \qquad \text{(sample size).}$$

2. Now obtain the standard error of the mean:

$$se_{\bar{x}} = s/\sqrt{n} \qquad = 4.1/\sqrt{174}$$

$$= 4.1/13.19 = 0.311 \text{ days.}$$

---

* Strictly we should have considered using the small population correction when calculating the standard deviation of the sampling distributions in Chapter 8, at least for the samples size 100, which were 8% of the population. The correction would have made a marginal difference in the two ranges of values theoretically containing 95% and 99% respectively of the samples.

3. If appropriate calculate the small population correction. Suppose the sample was drawn from a population size 1,608:

$$N = 1{,}608 \quad \text{(population size)}$$

$$\text{Correction} = \sqrt{\frac{N - n}{N - 1}} = \sqrt{\frac{1608 - 174}{1608 - 1}} = \sqrt{\frac{1434}{1607}}$$

$$= \sqrt{0.892} \quad = 0.945.$$

4. Multiply the original standard error (0.311) by the correction (0.945), to get an adjusted standard error, 0.294 days.
5. The 95% confidence limits are:

$$\bar{x} \pm 1.96 \times se_{\bar{x}}$$
$$19.2 \pm 1.96 \times 0.294*$$
$$19.2 \pm 0.58$$

18.62 days to 19.78 days or 18.6 to 19.8 days.
[Note the convention that the lower value of the range is given before the upper value.]
6. If requiring 99% confidence limits, these are

$$\bar{x} \pm 2.58 \times se_{\bar{x}}$$
$$19.2 \pm 2.58 \times 0.294$$
$$19.2 \pm 0.76$$

18.44 days to 19.96 days or 18.4 to 20.0 days.
7. Finally, for 99.9% confidence limits:

$$\bar{x} \pm 3.3 \times se_{\bar{x}}$$
$$19.2 \pm 3.3 \times 0.294$$
$$19.2 \pm 0.97$$

18.23 days to 20.17 days or 18.2 days to 20.2 days.

10.6　Estimating the Mean of Small Samples

Discussions so far have been about what are, technically, 'large samples'. The dividing line between large and small samples is taken at 30. Samples of 30 or under are treated as small samples.

The theoretical sampling distribution of small samples approximates to the Student-t or t distribution.[†] The dividing line of 30 between small

---

　*Remember the order of arithmetical processes as set out in the Mathematical Note. Multiply (1.96 × 0.294) before subtracting or adding.
　[†] The title Student-t derives from a pseudonym used by W S Gossett when he published his studies of the distribution in 1908.

and large samples is used because for sample sizes over 30, the normal and t distributions are very close, and it is therefore possible to use the normal distribution which is independent of sample size. The t distribution takes into account the sample size through 'degrees of freedom'. The number of degrees of freedom in the calculation of t is $(n - 1)$, where n is sample size.*

The t distribution has a slighly wider 'spread' than the normal distribution, so t values are higher than z values for the same probability, and t values increase as sample size declines. Since the smaller the sample size, the larger the standard error of the mean ($s/\sqrt{n}$), the net effect for a very small sample may be that confidence limits are so wide that meaningful conclusions are not possible. A table of the distribution of t is at the Appendix Table 2. It shows values of t for given probability levels for each degree of freedom from 1 to 30.

Suppose the group of dermatology patients whose mean length of stay in hospital we were studying (section 5 above) was only 25 in number.

1. The basic information is now:

$$\bar{x} = 19.2 \text{ days} \qquad \text{(sample mean)}$$

$$s = 4.1 \text{ days} \qquad \text{(sample standard deviation)}$$

$$n = 25 \text{ patients} \qquad \text{(sample size)}$$

2. The standard error is:

$$se_{\bar{x}} = s/\sqrt{n} = 4.1/\sqrt{25} = 4.1/5 = 0.82 \text{ days}$$

This is noticeably higher than for the sample of 174 patients (0.311 days).

3. The small population correction would not help. The percentage of the population sampled is only 1.6% and the factor is 0.993. We can ignore it.

4. From the t table we obtain the value of t corresponding to 24 degrees of freedom and 0.05 probability (2.064).[†]

---

*Degrees of freedom measure the number of ways in which data can vary given the restrictions imposed by the nature of the computation. In the calculation of s, the standard deviation, differences are taken from the mean. But their sum is always zero. So if $(n - 1)$ differences are already known, the final difference is automatically determined. One degree of freedom is lost. We start with n degrees of freedom (sample size) and therefore end up with $(n - 1)$ degrees of freedom for t.

[†] We have already referred to the area between the confidence limits being 0.95 or 95% of the total area of the normal curve. The probability 0.05 refers to the sum of the areas in the two symmetrical *tails* of the t distribution, and is the fraction of area (0.05 or 5%) outside the confidence limits. The equivalent of 99% confidence limits is probability 0.01, and of 99.9% confidence limits is probability 0.001.

5. The 95% confidence limits are

$$\bar{x} \pm 2.064 \times se_{\bar{x}}$$

$$19.2 \pm 2.064 \times 0.82$$

$$19.2 \pm 1.69$$

17.51 days to 20.89 days or 17.5 to 20.9 days.

6. These confidence limits are much wider than for the large sample of 174 patients (18.6 to 19.8 days). Wider limits also would be obtained for 99% confidence limits ($t = 2.797$) or 99.9% confidence limits ($t = 3.745$).

10.7   Estimating the Population Percentage

Sample means are derived from parametric data, interval data; percentages can be derived from any data, parametric or non-parametric, whether interval, ordinal or nominal. A percentage of a group represents the fraction of members of that group which possess a particular characteristic. Despite their different sources, there are circumstances in which means and percentages can be treated similarly. This applies not only to estimating population percentages, but also to tests concerning two percentages (Chapters 11 and 12).

Given a single sample percentage we can use this to estimate the percentage in the population. Suppose a single sample, size 100, drawn from the population of hospital dentists contain 47% whose age is under 40 years. We use the sample 47% both as the 'best estimate' of the percentage aged under 40 years in the population, and to calculate the standard deviation of the binomial distribution which is the standard error of the percentage.

Using algebraic notation,

$$p = 47\%\qquad\qquad\text{(sample percentage)}$$

$$n = 100\qquad\qquad\text{(sample size)}$$

$$se_p = \sqrt{\frac{p\%(100 - p)\%}{n}}\qquad\text{(standard error of percentage)}$$

$$= \sqrt{\frac{47 \times 53}{100}} = \sqrt{\frac{2{,}491}{100}}$$

$$= \sqrt{24.91} = 4.99\%.$$

The small population correction (see section 4 above) is 0.959, giving an adjusted standard error of 4.79%. The 95% confidence limits for the percentage of all hospital dentists (population) who are under 40 years of age will be:

$$p \pm 1.96 \times se_p$$

$$47 \pm 1.96 \times 4.79$$

$$47 \pm 9.39$$

$$37.61\% \text{ to } 56.39\% \text{ or } 37.6\% \text{ to } 56.4\%.$$

Note that the range of values does contain the population percentage which we know to be 51.90%.

Similarly we can obtain 99% confidence limits:

$$p \pm 2.58 \times se_p$$

$$47 \pm 2.58 \times 4.79$$

$$47 \pm 12.36$$

$$34.64\% \text{ to } 59.35\% \text{ or } 34.6\% \text{ to } 59.4\%$$

and 99.9% confidence limits:

$$p \pm 3.3 \times se_p$$

$$47 \pm 3.3 \times 4.79$$

$$47 \pm 15.81$$

$$31.19\% \text{ to } 62.81\% \text{ or } 31.2\% \text{ to } 62.8\%.$$

The approximation of the distribution of sample percentages to the normal curve holds provided the *number* of sample units with the measured characteristic is at least 5. If fewer than 5 sample units have the characteristic, we should not attempt to obtain confidence limits. The solution would be to take replicated samples to increase overall sample size. This would increase the number of sample units with the measured characteristic and thereby eliminate the problem.

10.8   A Reminder on Sample Size

The square root of sample size is *always* in the denominator of any standard error. Thus sample size has a major effect on the standard error. Larger sample sizes produce smaller standard errors.

We can improve on accuracy by increasing sample size, but the returns on so doing fall off rapidly. Standard error reduces in line with the *square root* of sample size. Doubling sample size from 100 to 200 will reduce standard error by approximately 30% i.e. by a factor of $1/\sqrt{2}$ ($=0.707$). To *halve* standard error means *quadrupling* sample size (the factor would be $1/\sqrt{4} = 0.5$). The cost of the sample size chosen must always be taken into account when designing research. A large sample size may be counter-productive if its high cost is met by economies which reduce accuracy elsewhere by more than the gain in statistical accuracy from the large sample size. A careful balancing act is required.

The confidence limits for the population percentage in section 7 above are very wide, the effect of using what is a small sample ($n = 100$). The standard error of the percentage is determined by the sample percentage and the sample size. It is a maximum when $p = 50\%$. With sample size 100, the maximum possible standard error is 5%. The standard error declines for either higher or lower values of p. For example, with sample size 100, if $p = 20\%$ (or 80%), the standard error is 4%; if $p = 10\%$ (or 90%), the standard error is 3%.

We should think carefully about the size of sample needed against the accuracy required in research results. This is particularly important for estimates of population percentages for which confidence limits can be quite wide. A method of working out a target sample size for a given degree of accuracy in sample percentages is set out in the note following.

Note on calculating target sample size for percentages. The highest value of a standard error will occur for sample percentages of 50%. If 95% confidence limits on estimates of about 50% are to be accurate at $\pm 5\%$, a range of 45% to 55%:

$$5 = 1.96 \times se_p$$

and

$$se_p = \sqrt{\frac{50 \times 50}{n}}$$

where n is the target sample size.

So,

$$5 = 1.96 \times \sqrt{\frac{2,500}{n}}$$

Squaring both sides of the equation:

$$5^2 = 1.96^2 \times \frac{2,500}{n}$$

and rearranging it:

$$n = \frac{3.84 \times 2,500}{25} = 384$$

In this example therefore, we would target the sample at 350 to 400 units.

The calculation above can be adapted for other degrees of accuracy, and for relating accuracy to other percentages, so providing the target sample size. A useful device.*

_____

For Reflection

Much data can be looked upon as being sample data. In particular, any data collected over a limited period of time is a sample of ongoing information, and is subject to chance error.

Estimates derived from samples are always subject to sampling error. This can apply in a wide variety of situations, whether looking at sick absences of staff, attendances at out-patient clinics, length of in-patient stay, recovery rates of patients, length of treatment to specific recovery, age or sex of patients registered for particular treatments, incidence of particular conditions. We must accept the possibility of error and make use of confidence limits on estimates.

Estimating the population parameter from the single sample leads to examining the relationship between a sample and a given population, and between two samples. Does a particular sample (mean or percentage) come from a known population? Is there a real difference between two sample results, not simply attributable to sampling error? These questions are considered in Chapters 11 and 12 following.

10.9   Summary

- You have now achieved a means of estimating a population parameter (mean or percentage) given information on a single sample only;
- you understand about the standard error as the measure of error arising from taking samples, and which is fundamental to interpreting research based on samples;
- starting with the single sample statistic as the 'best estimate' of the population parameter, you can obtain confidence limits as a range of values within which you are confident the population mean (or percentage) will fall. Your confidence is expressed in probability terms, and reflects the reliability of the statistical technique you are using;

_____

* The general expression is:

$$n = \frac{(z\text{-value for the chosen probability})^2 \times [p\%(100 - p)\%]}{(\text{acceptable error})^2}$$

where n is the target sample size, p is the target percentage to which the the error measurement is related, the z value is that selected to correspond to the confidence limits (1.96 for 95% confidence limits), and the acceptable error is the percentage error we will accept on the target percentage.

- the most commonly quoted are 95% confidence limits (probability of population parameter lying within this range is 0.95), but 99% and 99.9% confidence limits are also used;
- you are able to follow models for the basic method of calculation as shown in sections 5 and 7.

Further Reading

Discussions of the problems of estimation from sample results are to be found in:

Freund J E and Williams F J (1970 2nd edn) *Modern Business Statistics* Chapter 9. Bath: Pitman.

Hoel P G and Jessen R J (1977 2nd edn) *Basic Statistics for Business and Economics* Chapter 7. New York: Wiley.

Ott L, Larson R F and Meandenhall W (1983 3rd edn) *Statistics: A Tool for the Social Sciences* Chapter 6. Boston, Mass: Duxbury Press.

Reichman W J (1964) *Use and Abuse of Statistics* Chapter 15. London: Penguin.

A Little Practice

1. The mean cost of a random sample of 2,000 courses of dental treatment in 1990 was £30.5 per course with standard deviation £4.9. Obtain the 95% and 99% confidence limits for the mean cost of all courses of dental treatment in 1990.

2. The mean length of stay for a random sample of 169 maternity patients who gave birth in a particular hospital in 1990 was 4.9 days with standard deviation 1.1 day. Use this information to obtain 95% confidence limits for the mean length of stay of all maternity patients in the hospital in 1990.

3. The mean number of days for completion of a particular course of treatment at a hospital for a random sample of 92 out-patients was 45.4 days with standard deviation 4.3 days. Obtain the 99.9% confidence limits for the mean length of treatment for all out-patients.

4. Out of a random sample of 354 patients treated for a particular condition, 75% left hospital by the 5th day after completion of treatment. What are the 95% confidence limits for the percentage of all patients leaving hospital by the 5th day after completion of treatment?

5. A random sample of 150 patients on a general practitioner's list were asked if they would prefer a later Friday evening surgery or a Saturday morning surgery. Ninety-three said they would prefer the late evening

surgery. What are the 99% confidence limits for the percentage of all patients on the general practitioner's list who would prefer the late evening surgery? (Remember to calculate the *percentage* of patients preferring the late evening surgery first.)

6. Out of 135 student nurses in a new intake in a particular hospital, 97 decided to live in hospital accommodation. On the basis that the group can be looked upon as a random sample of all student nurses entering training at the hospital, what are the 95% confidence limits for the percentage of all student nurses preferring to live in hospital accommodation? (Again, remember to calculate the *percentage* of the intake preferring hospital accommodation. Take your percentage to 2 decimal places as you are going to use it in further calculations.)

11

Significance Tests:
The Sample Statistic and
the Population Parameter

11.1 Sample and Population Means—Large Samples

In Chapter 10 we learnt to estimate the population parameter from a single sample statistic, either a mean or a percentage, and provide a measure of error on that estimate. This leads to considering whether a single sample could have come from a population with a known mean or percentage. The population parameter can be based on known information, or be hypothesised.

Suppose we are studying the time lapse between the commencement of a course of new treatment for a skin condition, and the achievement of a specific measurable improvement. Past records of the previous treatment show a mean time lapse of 43.6 days (population mean). The new treatment, using a sample of 73 patients, leads to a mean time lapse of 40.3 days with standard deviation 9.5 days. The difference between the means is not great—3.3 days. Does the new treatment represent an improvement? Or is it possible that the apparent improvement is due to sampling error?

We tackle the problem by setting up a Null Hypothesis of no difference between the two mean values, that the real difference between the sample mean (40.3 days) and the population mean (43.6 days) is zero, that the observed difference is due to sampling error.

From normal curve theory, if we take many samples from a population, and record the differences between each sample mean and the population mean, these observed differences will be distributed normally with mean of zero and standard deviation equal to the standard error of the mean. With a single sample, we can look at the difference between the sample mean and the population mean and establish the probability that a difference of this magnitude could occur through sampling error.

We convert the difference into a z-value (the standard unit of Chapter 7.6) by dividing it by the standard error of the mean. Using the normal curve area table we can establish the probability with which any z-value could occur and therefore whether or not the observed difference could be due to sampling error:

$$z = \frac{\text{observed difference}}{\text{appropriate standard error}}$$

A useful approach with wide application is to think of this as the ratio between the empirical difference and the theoretical difference. Common-sense tells us that the larger this ratio, the more likely the difference is to be real and not due to sampling error.

The data is $\mu = 43.6$ days, $\bar{x} = 40.3$ days, $s = 9.5$ days, $n = 73$ patients.

First calculate the standard error using the sample standard deviation as 'best estimate' of the population standard deviation:

$$z = \frac{\bar{x} - \mu}{se_{\bar{x}}} \quad \text{where } se_{\bar{x}} = s/\sqrt{n}$$

$$se_{\bar{x}} = 9.5/\sqrt{73} = 1.11 \text{ days}$$

Then

$$z = \frac{40.3 - 43.6}{1.11} = \frac{-3.3}{1.11} = -2.97*$$

We require a criterion for deciding whether or not the sample has come from the population. What we use is a probability of being **wrong** if we say the sample does not come from the population. The probability commonly used is 0.05. We look to the value of z at which the area in the two tails together is 0.05 (5%) of total area, so excluding the extreme 5% of samples. The z value is 1.96, which corresponds to the factor for 95% confidence limits. This is shown in Figure 11.1 with the area for rejecting the Null Hypothesis hatched. We could choose a more stringent probability, 0.01 ($z = 2.58$) or 0.001 ($z = 3.3$). But the use of 0.05 probability as a criterion has a long history and in practice works well. As part of the conclusions we look at calculated z against the more stringent test levels.

On the data, $|z| = 2.97$,[†] and $|z| > z_{0.05}$ (1.96).[‡] On the criterion of 0.05 probability, we would reject the Null Hypothesis and say that the sample does not come from the population, that there is a real difference between the mean lapses of time for the old and new treatments. We can be

---

* The negative sign of z indicates that the sample mean is smaller than the population mean, and that the z value is in the negative half of the curve. Because the curve is symmetrical, areas related to negative values are the same as areas related to the corresponding positive values. The areas themselves are always positive.

† The upright parallel lines round z means 'arithmetic value of z, irrespective of sign' thus ignoring the direction (+ or −) of z. It is simpler to look at calculated z in this way in relation to the standard normal curve values.

‡ The symbol > means 'greater than' the value following. The subscript indicates the probability level of the z-value.

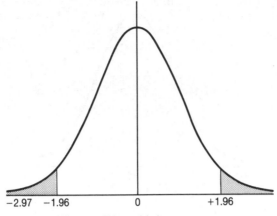

Figure 11.1

confident in asserting that the new treatment leads to slightly speedier improvement. Note that we could reject the Null Hypothesis at 0.01 probability ($z_{0.01} = 2.58$) strengthening the conclusion, but not at 0.001 probability ($z_{0.001} = 3.3$).

As another example, research in a particular hospital concerns the mean length of in-patient stay for a surgical procedure. Previous records show a mean of 8.8 days (population mean); in a current year, the mean length of in-patient stay for 40 patients is 9.2 days with standard deviation 3.2 days. Has the mean length of stay risen? Or could the difference be due to sampling error?

Here $\mu = 8.8$ days, $\bar{x} = 9.2$ days, $s = 3.2$ days, $n = 40$ patients:

$$se_{\bar{x}} = 3.2/\sqrt{40} = 3.2/6.32 = 0.51 \text{ days}$$

$$z = \frac{\bar{x} - \mu}{se_{\bar{x}}} = \frac{9.2 - 8.8}{0.51} = \frac{0.4}{0.51} = 0.78$$

Since $|z| = 0.78$, $|z| < z_{0.05}$ (1.96) we cannot reject the Null Hypothesis.* Can we accept it?

11.2 An Important Digression on Probability

Reverting to the first example in section 1, consider the probability of an observed difference being due to sampling error. Here $|z| = 2.97$; the area in the two symmetrical tails of the sampling distribution represents the probability of a difference as big as that observed ($\bar{x} - \mu$) arising through sampling error. This is shown in Figure 11.2.

---

* The symbol < means 'less than' the value following.

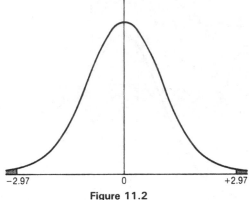

Figure 11.2

Look at the normal curve area table, and find the area in the two tails for $z = 2.97$. This is 0.0030.* For the calculated value of z there is a probability of only 0.003 (or 0.3%) that the observed difference could have been due to sampling error, and a probability of $[1 - 0.003 = 0.997]$, that the difference is 'real'. We are therefore very confident in saying that there is a difference not due to sampling error. It is called a 'statistically significant difference'.

In the second example from section 1, the calculated value is $|z| = 0.78$ and the Null Hypothesis was not rejected. What more could we have concluded? Do we accept the Null Hypothesis? Look again at the normal curve area table and the probability of getting a difference the size of that observed through sampling error. This time it is 0.4354 (43.5%)[†] and is represented by the hatched areas in Figure 11.3. We would be willing to accept the Null Hypothesis, not because $|z| < z_{0.05}$ (1.96), but because the Null Hypothesis has a substantial probability of being correct.

Whatever the conclusion, we run the risk of making a mistake; that the correct situation is the reverse of the conclusion. The relationship between the real situation and the conclusion is set out below.

	Test conclusion	
Real situation	Sample is from population	Sample is not from population
Sample is from population	CORRECT NH not rejected	False conclusion Type I error
Sample is not from population	False conclusion Type II error	CORRECT NH rejected

---

*Area 0 to $z = 2.97$ is 0.4985, so the area in the single tail is $[0.5 - 0.4985 = 0.0015]$. This is doubled to give the area in the two tails as 0.0030.

[†]Area 0 to $z = 0.78$ is 0.2823. The area in the single tail is $[0.5 - 0.2823 = 0.2177]$, giving the area in the two tails as 0.4354.

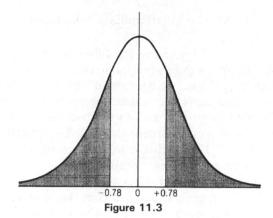

Figure 11.3

The four possible conclusions from a significance test are:

1. that the sample is from the population and the test confirms it. A CORRECT result;
2. that the sample is not from the population when in fact it is. This is a FALSE conclusion, known as a Type I error, the error of rejecting a true (null) hypothesis;
3. that the sample is from the population when it is not. This too is a FALSE conclusion and is a Type II error, the error of accepting a false (null) hypothesis;
4. that the sample is not from the population, and the test confirms this. A CORRECT result.

When rejecting the Null Hypothesis at 0.05 probability, we are concentrating on the Type I error, and ignoring the Type II error. Why do this? If we make a Type I error we assert that there is a real difference when there is not. It is essential to hold the risk of this error at a low level, because important decisions may depend on the conclusion. In the first example above, we would want to be reasonably confident that the new treatment is an improvement on the old before introducing it. Changing treatments, introducing new drugs, we need to know that this is the right decision. In general it is more hazardous to conclude a real difference exists when it does not, than to conclude that the difference is due to sampling error when the reverse is the case (Type II error). In order to be confident the conclusion will stand, we use a test level with a low probability of being wrong if we conclude a difference exists. In deciding what test level to use, we accept a probability of being wrong in the conclusion. If 0.05 probability represents too high a risk, we can test at 0.01 probability ($z_{0.01} = 2.58$) or 0.001 probability ($z_{0.001} = 3.3$). The decision as to the test level to use will depend on circumstances, the importance of potential change, the existence of other research results etc.

11.3   The Indeterminate Conclusion

We have looked at results leading to the rejection or the acceptance of a Null Hypothesis. There is a third situation to consider. Suppose $|z| = 1.73$. This is less than $z_{0.05}$ (1.96), so we cannot reject the Null Hypothesis. Looking at the normal curve area table, the probability that the sample comes from the population (the area in the two tails) is 0.1032 (approx. 10%). We would be unwise to accept the Null Hypothesis since it has a probability of only 1 in 10 of being true, and a probability of 9 in 10 of being false. This is an indeterminate result.

We should not accept the Null Hypothesis if $|z|$ is fairly close to the test value of 1.96. As a general guide accept the Null Hypothesis when $|z|$ is about 1 or a lower value. The alternative to rejecting a Null Hypothesis is not necessarily to accept it, but to say that no firm conclusion is possible. What can we do in that situation? We seek more information, more samples. Replicating the study, effectively increasing sample size and reducing the standard error, provides prospects of reaching a firm conclusion.

11.4   Sample and Population Means—Small Samples

If the first sample of patients in section 1 had been small, 30 or less, we would have calculated the t-statistic, not a z-value. This is comparable to using t in deriving confidence limits for the means of small samples (Chapter 10.6).

If the research had covered only 28 patients:

$$\mu = 43.6 \text{ days}, \quad \bar{x} = 40.3 \text{ days}, \quad s = 9.5 \text{ days}, \quad n = 28 \text{ patients}$$

$$se_{\bar{x}} = s/\sqrt{n} = 9.5/\sqrt{28} = 9.5/5.29 = 1.79$$

$$t = \frac{\bar{x} - \mu}{se_{\bar{x}}}$$

$$= \frac{40.3 - 43.6}{1.79} = \frac{-3.3}{1.79} = -1.84$$

From the table of t, the value of $t_{0.05}$ for 27 (28 − 1) degrees of freedom is 2.052. From the data $|t| = 1.84$, so we cannot reject the Null Hypothesis. Since t is quite high (the probability that the sample is not from the population hypothesised is approximately 0.9), we would not accept the Null Hypothesis. It is a case for more information, for an increase in the overall sample size by replicating the research with another group of patients.

11.5 Sample and Population Percentages

Exactly the same arguments apply to percentages. Considering the new and old treatments for the skin condition, we could study the rapidity of recovery by recording the number of patients in whom the improvement occurred within 45 days. For the previous treatment, records show that this was 64.75%. Amongst the 73 patients experiencing the new treatment, 49 (67.12%) improved within 45 days.

The data is

$$\theta = 64.75\%, \quad p = 67.12\%, \quad n = 73 \text{ patients}$$

$$z = \frac{\text{observed difference}}{\text{appropriate standard error}} = \frac{p - \theta}{se_p}$$

$$se_p = \sqrt{\frac{\theta\%(100 - \theta)\%}{n}} * = \sqrt{\frac{64.75 \times 35.25}{73}} = 5.59\%$$

$$z = \frac{67.12 - 64.75}{5.59} = \frac{2.37}{5.59} = 0.42$$

$|z| < z_{0.05}$ (1.96), so we cannot reject the Null Hypothesis. It is very low indeed. The probability that the new treatment has *not* led to an increase in the percentage improving within 45 days is approximately 0.67; the probability that it *has* led to an improvement is 0.33—two to one *against* an increase in the percentage showing improvement within 45 days.

The conclusion must be to accept the Null Hypothesis and to say that there is no change in the percentage improving within 45 days. For some whose improvement is slow, the new treatment appears to be no advantage over the old. Perhaps we should seek to identify the characteristics of those patients who appear to have benefited from the new treatment? Perhaps for some the old treatment might be just as effective as the new or even better? We would need to carry out further research to investigate these points.

11.6 Summary

In this chapter you have looked at an area of statistics very important to the interpretation of research results based on samples:

- you have examined the difference between a sample statistic (mean or percentage) and a population parameter in order to infer whether the sample is likely to have been drawn from that population;

---

*We have a population percentage, so are able to use it in the calculation of the standard error.

- you have been introduced to the use of the Null Hypothesis, and to the error involved in either rejecting or accepting it;
- you are aware that an indeterminate situation is possible, and that this can be resolved by further research.

Note. This is a halfway point. Chapter 12 completes the study of significance tests, and in section 4 includes a formal example as a model for the process of computation and the interpretation of results. It is worth returning to the discussions of concepts in both chapters once the mechanics are mastered.

The Further Reading and Practice sections at the end of Chapter 12 cover both chapters.

12

Significance Tests:
The Difference Between
Two Sample Statistics

12.1 Two Sample Means—Large Samples

In Chapter 11 we learnt how to conduct a significance test using the results from a single sample and a known (or hypothesised) population parameter. Often we are not comparing a sample statistic with a population parameter, but are studying two samples. Is there a real difference between the two samples, other than can be accounted for by sampling error? Do the samples come from the same population, from similar populations? The alternative is that the difference between the sample results is real, that they come from different populations.

Many research situations take this form. A study comparing two groups of patients receiving different treatments, research into length of in-patient stay in different hospitals, comparison between men and women in the incidence of disease, change between years in the number of cases registered for a particular condition, research into wastage rates of student nurses training for different sections of the register or at different hospitals, can be expressed as a comparison between two samples.

With two populations, we can draw many pairs of samples, calculate means, and measure the difference between means of each pair of samples. What would be the characteristics of a frequency distribution created from these differences? * The distribution would approximate to a normal distribution with a mean of $(\mu_1 - \mu_2)$, the difference between the population means μ_1 and μ_2. Its standard deviation, known as the standard error of the difference between two sample means, is

$$\sqrt{\frac{\sigma_1^2}{n_1} + \frac{\sigma_2^2}{n_2}}$$

---

* Taking samples in order drawn, some of the differences would be positive, some of them negative, and the positive/negative sign would be retained in the frequency distribution.

where σ_1 and σ_2 are the standard deviations of the two populations, and n_1, n_2 the sample sizes.* If the pairs of samples come from the same population, $\mu_1 = \mu_2$, and $[\mu - \mu_2 = 0]$.

In research we commonly have two samples which may or may not come from the same population. A Null Hypothesis that there is no difference between two sample statistics implies that the samples are from the same or similar populations, and that the mean difference between the sample statistics is zero.

As for estimating the population mean through confidence limits and examining the difference between sample and population means, we do not know the standard deviation of the population(s) from which the samples are drawn, so use the sample standard deviations to obtain a 'best estimate' for the standard error of the difference between two sample means. The standard error is:

$$se_{\bar{x}_1 - \bar{x}_2} = \sqrt{\frac{s_1^2}{n_1} + \frac{s_2^2}{n_2}}$$

We have now established the principles upon which to operate.

Consider the example of treatment for a particular skin condition, with an ongoing research study comparing new and old treatments. Patients are studied in two groups; Group A is experiencing the new treatment, Group B the old treatment. The outcome is comparing the groups in terms of the mean number of days elapsing until a specific improvement has occurred. We have the following results:

	Group A	Group B
Mean length of treatment	$\bar{x}_1 = 40.3$ days	$\bar{x}_2 = 45.4$ days
Standard deviation	$s_1 = 9.5$ days	$s_2 = 10.1$ days
Sample size	$n_1 = 73$ patients	$n_2 = 125$ patients

The Null Hypothesis is that there is no real difference between the two sample means, that the treatments lead to identical results. The Null Hypothesis is to be tested at 0.05 probability.[†] We calculate z, and reject the Null Hypothesis if $|z| \geq z_{0.05}$ (1.96).[‡] Exactly the same arguments about conclusions apply here as in Chapter 11.

The standard error of the difference between the sample means is:

$$\sqrt{\frac{s_1^2}{n_1} + \frac{s_2^2}{n_2}} = \sqrt{\frac{9.5^2}{73} + \frac{10.1^2}{125}}$$

---

* To distinguish between the two samples, subscripts indicating sample one and sample two are added to the standard forms of algebraic notation.

[†] As before, we use 0.05 probability as a basic test level, then examine the effect of using more stringent probability levels.

[‡] The symbol $\geq$ means 'greater than or equal to' the value following.

$$= \sqrt{\frac{90.25}{73} + \frac{102.01}{125}} = \sqrt{1.236 + 0.816}$$

$$= \sqrt{2.052} = 1.43 \text{ days}$$

As in Chapter 11, we calculate z:

$$z = \frac{\text{observed difference}}{\text{appropriate standard error}} = \frac{\bar{x}_1 - \bar{x}_2}{se_{\bar{x}_1 - \bar{x}_2}}$$

$$= \frac{40.3 - 45.4}{1.43} = \frac{-5.1}{1.43} = -3.57$$

The result is a $|z|$ value that (in magnitude) not only exceeds $z_{0.05}$ (1.96) but also exceeds the more stringent test levels of $z_{0.01}$ (2.58) and $z_{0.001}$ (3.3). The probability that the difference between the two sample means is due to sampling error is less than 0.001, less than one in a thousand. We are therefore very confident in rejecting the Null Hypothesis and affirming that there is a real difference in the results from the two treatments, a difference not due to sampling error. The new treatment leads to a reduced mean lapse of time to specific improvement.

12.2   Two Sample Means—Small Samples

The argument about the distribution of the difference between the means of two small samples is exactly the same as for large samples. The distribution to which the difference between the means of small samples approximate is the t distribution (see Chapter 10.6), and we calculate that statistic. The standard error of the difference between the means of two small samples is:

$$se_{\bar{x}_1 - \bar{x}_2} = \sqrt{\frac{(n_1 - 1)s_1^2 + (n_2 - 1)s_2^2}{(n_1 - 1) + (n_2 - 1)} \left(\frac{1}{n_1} + \frac{1}{n_2}\right)}$$

where s_1, s_2 are the standard deviations of the two samples, and n_1, n_2 the sample sizes. The degrees of freedom are $[(n_1 - 1) + (n_2 - 1)]$ or $[n_1 + n_2 - 2]$.

Data from the new treatment (Group A) and the old treatment (Group B) provides the following information:

	Group A	Group B
Mean length of treatment	$\bar{x}_1 = 40.3$ days	$\bar{x}_2 = 45.4$ days
Standard deviation	$s_1 = 9.5$ days	$s_2 = 10.1$ days
Number of patients	$n_1 = 16$ patients	$n_2 = 12$ patients

$$se_{\bar{x}_1 - \bar{x}_2} = \sqrt{\frac{(15 \times 9.5^2) + (11 \times 10.1^2)}{15 + 11} \left(\frac{1}{16} + \frac{1}{12}\right)}$$

$$= \sqrt{\frac{15 \times 90.25 + 11 \times 102.01}{26} \times (0.0625 + 0.0833)}$$

$$= \sqrt{\frac{1,352.75 + 1,122.11}{26} \times 0.1458}$$

$$= \sqrt{\frac{2,475.86}{26} \times 0.1458} = \sqrt{95.23 \times 0.1458}$$

$$= \sqrt{13.88} = 3.73 \text{ days}$$

$$t = \frac{\text{observed difference}}{\text{appropriate standard error}}$$

$$= \frac{\bar{x}_1 - \bar{x}_2}{se_{\bar{x}_1 - \bar{x}_2}} = \frac{40.3 - 45.4}{3.73} = \frac{-5.1}{3.73} = -1.37$$

From the table of t, $t_{0.05}$ for $[(n_1 + n_2 - 2) = 26]$ degrees of freedom is 2.056. We cannot reject the Null Hypothesis; $|t| < t_{0.05}$. The probability of $|t| \geq 1.37$ occurring through sampling error is approximately 0.2, a 1 in 5 probability. In view of this low probability, we might hesitate to accept the Null Hypothesis, view the result as indeterminate, and seek to study further samples.

12.3   Two Sample Percentages

We can test for a significant difference between two sample percentages, p_1 and p_2. A series of differences between pairs of percentages sampled from different populations $(p_1 - p_2)$ would form a frequency distribution approximating to a normal distribution with a mean percentage of $(\theta_1 - \theta_2)$, and a standard deviation, the standard error of the difference between sample percentages, of:

$$se_{p_1 - p_2} = \sqrt{\frac{\theta_1\%(100 - \theta_1)\%}{n_1} + \frac{\theta_2\%(100 - \theta_2)\%}{n_2}}$$

where θ_1 and θ_2 are the percentages in the two populations, and n_1 and n_2 are the two sample sizes.

Having no information about population percentages, the sample percentages are used as 'best estimates' of the percentages in the two populations. As with two sample means, the basis of the Null Hypothesis is that the sample percentages are from the same or similar populations, so $[(p_1 - p_2) = 0]$.

We could look at the groups of patients (Group A new treatment; Group B old treatment) in terms of the percentages of patients who made a specific improvement within 45 days.

	Group A	Group B
Number of patients improving within 45 days	$x_1 = 49$	$x_2 = 79$
Sample size	$n_1 = 73$	$n_2 = 125$
Percentage of patients improving (x/n)	$p_1 = 67.12\%$	$p_2 = 63.20\%$

$$z = \frac{p_1 - p_2}{se_{p_1-p_2}}$$

and,

$$se_{p_1-p_2} = \sqrt{\frac{p_1\%(100 - p_1)\%}{n_1} + \frac{p_2\%(100 - p_2)\%}{n_2}}$$

$$= \sqrt{\frac{67.12 \times 32.88}{73} + \frac{63.2 \times 36.8}{125}}$$

$$= \sqrt{\frac{2,206.91}{73} + \frac{2,325.76}{125}} = \sqrt{30.23 + 18.61}$$

$$= \sqrt{48.84} = 6.99\%$$

$$z = \frac{67.12 - 63.2}{6.99} = \frac{3.92}{6.99} = 0.56$$

Although there is a difference of nearly 4% between the two sample percentages, the z value at 0.56 is not only below 1.96 but is a very low value. The probability of this difference arising on account of sampling error is approximately 0.58, greater than 1 in 2. The observed difference is more likely to have arisen through the sampling process than to be due to a real difference between the two sample percentages. We would undoubtedly accept the Null Hypothesis. More research, possibly a redesigned research project, would be needed if we wished to pursue the question further.

12.4   Significance Test Calculations

Suitable illustrative examples have been included in the text in this and the preceding chapter. This is a good moment to pause, and to set out the formal steps in any significance test calculation and conclusion. We have covered four significance tests, each involving the difference between two values. They are:

1. Sample and population—means   Chapter 11.1, 11.4
2. Sample and population—percentages   Chapter 11.5
3. Two samples   —means   sections 1 and 2 above
4. Two samples   —percentages   section 3 above

Briefly the steps are (1) summarising the research information needed for the test; (2) stating the Null Hypothesis; (3) setting out the test criterion; (4) calculating z; (5) comparing calculated $|z|$ with the test value of z and deciding whether or not to reject the Null Hypothesis; (6) considering any possible further conclusions in extension of (5).

Using the data from section 1 for the formal process of a test between two sample means:*

1. Research on two groups of patients receiving different treatments for a particular skin condition examines the lapse of time between commencement of treatment and a specific improvement. For Group A (new treatment), consisting of 73 patients, the mean lapse of time is 40.3 days with standard deviation 9.5 days. For Group B (old treatment), 125 patients, the mean lapse of time is 45.4 days with standard deviation 10.1 days.
2. The Null Hypothesis is that there is no real difference between the mean lapse of time to specific improvement for Group A patients (40.3 days) and that for Group B patients (45.4 days); the observed difference is due to sampling error.
3. The Null Hypothesis is tested at 0.05 probability. Reject the Null Hypothesis if calculated $|z| \geq z_{0.05}$ (1.96).†
4. Set out the relevant information:

	Group A	Group B
Mean length of treatment	$\bar{x}_1 = 40.3$ days	$\bar{x}_2 = 45.4$ days
Standard deviation	$s_1 = 9.5$ days	$s_2 = 10.1$ days
Sample size	$n_1 = 73$ patients	$n_2 = 125$ patients

$$se_{\bar{x}_1-\bar{x}_2} = \sqrt{\frac{s_1^2}{n_1} + \frac{s_2^2}{n_2}} = \sqrt{\frac{9.5^2}{73} + \frac{10.1^2}{125}} = \sqrt{\frac{90.25}{73} + \frac{102.01}{125}}$$

$$= \sqrt{1.236 + 0.816} = \sqrt{2.052} = 1.43$$

$$z = \frac{\text{observed difference}}{\text{appropriate standard error}} = \frac{\bar{x}_1 - \bar{x}_2}{se_{\bar{x}_1-\bar{x}_2}} = \frac{40.3 - 45.4}{1.43} = -3.57$$

---

* The same procedure is followed for others of the four significance tests.
† The criterion of $z_{0.05}$ (1.96) for testing the Null Hypothesis applies to large samples. Where small samples are involved calculate a t statistic and compare it with the value of $t_{0.05}$ for the appropriate degrees of freedom ($n_1 + n_2 - 2$). The same method then applies.

5. $|z| > z_{0.05}$ (1.96). We therefore reject the Null Hypothesis and conclude that there is a real difference between the mean lapses of time for the two sample groups. There is a statistically significant difference between the two means.

6. Looking at calculated $|z|$ (3.57) against more stringent test levels; $|z| > z_{0.01}$ (2.58) and $z_{0.001}$ (3.3). We can also reject the Null Hypothesis at 0.01 probability (a highly significant difference) and at 0.001 probability (a very highly significant difference). The new treatment is confirmed as more effective than the old.

7. Had the $|z|$ value been about 1.0 or less, we would have considered accepting the Null Hypothesis. For $|z|$ values above 1.0 but less than 1.96, careful consideration might lead to an indeterminate conclusion. Further research might lead to firm conclusions.

12.5   Sample Size With Two Samples

A final comment on sample size. As already noted, this has an important effect on the magnitude of the standard error. With two samples, their respective sizes are taken into account in the calculation of the standard error. It does not matter therefore, whether the samples are of approximately equal size or very different. For a research project comparing two groups, the results will be most efficient (minimum standard error, maximum likelihood of a significant difference) if the two groups are of approximately equal size.

12.6   One-Tailed Tests and Two-Tailed Tests

In this and the preceding chapter, significance tests have all been treated as two-tailed tests. The Null Hypothesis has focused on the absolute difference between the two measures, not on the direction of the difference, whether one measure is larger (or smaller) than the other. Some tests can be formulated as one-tailed tests; the question of new treatment leading to speedier recovery is such an example. Unless the evidence suggested that the new treatment might be better, we would not be investigating this through a significance test. In this situation we could be looking at the area in the single tail only as the test criterion. In a one-tailed test conducted at 0.05 probability, 5% of the area under the normal curve is in the single tail and $z_{0.05} = 1.65$. This is a less stringent test than the two-tailed test that we have used. One-tailed tests and two-tailed tests are not comparable. It is safer, and consistent, to use two-tailed tests. The Further Reading section includes texts which discuss this aspect.

12.7 A Word of Caution

The last two chapters have established a method of looking at a population and a sample or two samples, and deciding whether the difference between means or percentages is statistically significant or attributable to sampling error.

One swallow does not make a summer. One statistically significant difference, in isolation, must be viewed with caution. Significance tests, and statistically significant results, are part of the total scene. They should fit in and be consistent with other information. We would expect a pattern of statistically significant results, not one alone. The single statistically significant result is an indicator we should follow up, seek out other information, conduct other significance tests; it cannot be used on its own to indicate change or difference. Never forget that when testing at the 0.05 probability level, we expect to be wrong around 1 in 20 times when saying there is a statistically significant difference.

Significance tests are of wide application and are part of the total means of interpreting research results and other statistical information.

12.8 Summary

- You have achieved a method for establishing statistically significant differences between two sample measures;
- you have examined two sample means and two sample percentages to decide whether or not two samples have come from the same population;
- you can now decide whether any difference between means or percentages is statistically significant, or whether it is due to sampling error. This contributes to the tools available for examining and interpreting research results.

Section 4 above sets out a model for you to follow.

Further Reading

Caulcott E (1973) *Significance Tests* Chapter 5. London: Routledge and Kegan Paul. Chapter 6 contains a useful discussion on interpreting statistically significant differences.

Freund J E (1979 5th edn) *Modern Elementary Statistics* Chapter 10. London: Prentice-Hall.

Hoel P G and Jessen R J (1977 2nd edn) *Basic Statistics for Business and Economics* Chapter 8. New York: Wiley.

Ott L, Larson R F and Mendenhall W (1983 3rd edn) *Statistics: a Tool for the Social Sciences* Chapter 8. Boston, Mass: Duxbury Press.

A Little Practice

1. The mean age at entry to training for 163 student nurses starting training at Hospital A in a current year is 19.8 years with standard deviation 2.1 years. Previous records over several years show mean age at entry as 19.1 years. Does this suggest the mean age at entry to training at Hospital A is rising? (Is there a statistically significant difference between the mean age at entry currently and the previously established (population) mean age at entry?)

2. In a clinical trial, a new method of treatment is compared with the current method used. The new method leads to a standardised improvement in the 79 experimental group patients after a mean time lapse of 54.2 days, with standard deviation 5.5 days. Records for the current method of treatment show mean time lapse to standardised improvement of 58.7 days. Is the new method of treatment an improvement? (Test whether there is a statistically significant difference between the mean lapse of time for the experimental group and the previously established (population) mean time lapse for the current treatment.)

3. In England 34.9% of *all* general medical practitioners work in partnerships of 5 or more doctors. In a RHA A, 32.6% of a random sample of 450 general medical practitioners work in partnerships of 5 or more doctors. Do fewer doctors work in large partnerships in RHA A? (Is there a statistically significant difference between the percentage of general medical practitioners in England (population) in partnerships of 5 or more and the equivalent percentage in the sample from RHA A?)

4. At a particular hospital, records for previous years show that approximately 80% of student nurses have chosen to live in hospital accommodation. For intakes of nurses in a current year totalling 153 students, 110 decided to live in hospital accommodation. Does this suggest that the hospital's accommodation is less popular with student nurses? (Test whether there is a statistically significant difference between the previous percentage of student nurses living in hospital accommodation (population) and the percentage for the current year. Do not forget to calculate first the percentage for the current year.)

5. The mean number of patients on the lists of a random sample of 216 general medical practitioners in RHA A, is 2,012 with standard deviation 377 patients. In another RHA B, the mean size of list of a random sample of 354 general medical practitioners is 1,961 patients with standard deviation 315 patients. Are list sizes larger in RHA A compared with RHA B? [Is there a statistically significant difference between the mean list sizes in areas A and B?]

6. Random samples are taken from patients in two general surgical wards in a particular hospital. In Ward A the sample of 110 patients had a mean length of stay of 7.3 days with standard deviation 2.7 days. For the sample of 80 patients from Ward B, the mean length of stay was 6.6 days with standard deviation 2.5 days. Do patients from Ward A spend longer in hospital than those from Ward B? (Test whether there is a statistically significant difference between the mean length of stay for the two wards.)

7. At Hospital A, 89% of a random sample of 53 student nuses passed their final examination at the first attempt. At Hospital B, 91% of a random sample of 57 student nurses passed their final examination at the first attempt. Were nurses at Hospital A more successful than those at Hospital B? (Is there a statistically significant difference between the percentages passing at their first attempt at the two hospitals?)

8. In a drugs trial, a random sample of 213 patients were treated with a new drug and 182 were assessed as reaching a particular level of improvement within 45 days. A second random sample of 450 patients received conventional treatment, and of these 345 achieved the particular level of improvement within 45 days. Is the new drug an improvement on the conventional treatment? (Is there a statistically significant difference between the two sample groups in the percentages achieving the particular level of improvement within 45 days?)

13

Data Patterns:
The Chi-square Test

13.1 The Contingency Table

We have examined the relationship between two sample values (whether means or percentages), and have conducted significance tests to establish whether an observed difference between them is real or should be attributed to sampling error. Research often produces more elaborate sample data, a series of samples or sub-samples, demonstrating more complex patterns which require assessment. Data of this kind is shown in contingency tables. Here the same overall sample data is spread across two sets of attributes, for example, different lengths of time to recovery by age of patient. Is number of days to recovery contingent upon the age of the patient, is there an association between age of patient and number of days to recovery? Or is any apparent association no more than might arise on account of the sampling process? A contingency table sets out data in such a way that we can examine the possibility that one variable is contingent upon the other.

The chi-square test applies to non-parametric data. Parametric data (number of days to recovery, age of patient) may be converted into ordinal data by suitable grouping (see Table 13.1). A wide variety of non-parametric attributes (such as sex, socio-economic group, treatment given, severity of condition, satisfaction with care) can be subjected to this test. Although it is not overtly apparent, the chi-square test is dealing with differences between the percentage distributions of data across the sets of attributes. The test is very flexible in terms of the situations it can handle, and is very important when drawing conclusions from research studies based on several sample subgroups.

13.2 The Chi-square Test

Suppose a research project examining the relationship between age at commencement of treatment and the length of treatment for a particular skin condition involves 800 patients. For each patient we record age in years

at the commencement of treatment and the number of days from the start
of treatment until a specific improvement is achieved. At the end of the
research study the data obtained is set out in a contingency table.*

Table 13.1 Age of patient and length of time to specific improvement

Age in years of patient at commencement of treatment	Number of days from commencement of treatment to specific improvement			
	Under 25	25 to 49	50 and over	All patients
Under 30	175	120	65	360
30 and under 60	105	90	61	256
60 and over	20	90	74	184
All ages	300	300	200	800

The overall sample (800 cases), has been divided across three categories of
age, and three categories of number of days to specific improvement as
shown in Table 13.1. What would we expect if there is no association
between the age of the patient and the outcome of treatment?

Out of the total of 800 patients, 360 or 45% are aged under 30 years. If
there is no association between age and number of days to specific improvement, we would expect 45% of each of the three length of treatment groups
to be aged under 30 years. So in the first group who improved in under 25
days, we would expect 135 patients under 30 years; in the second group who
improved in 25 to 49 days, 135 patients are expected to be under 30 years;
and in the third group who improved in 50 or more days, 90 patients are
expected to be under 30 years.

Turning to patients 30 and under 60 years, these are 32% of all patients.
Applying the same argument, we would expect 32% of each length of
treatment group to be 30 and under 60 years. So for patients improving in
less than 25 days, 96 are expected to be 30 and under 60 years; for those
improving in 25 to 49 days, 96 are expected to be 30 to 60 years; for those
improving in 50 or more days, 64 are expected to be in this age-group.

The final age-group, over 60 years, is 23% of all patients. We would
expect 23% of those improving in less than 25 days (69 patients), 23% of
those improving in 25 to 49 days (69 patients) and 23% of those improving
in 50 or more days (46 patients) to be in the age-group over 60 years.[†]

Expectation here is on the basis that there is no association between
age and lapse of time to specific improvement, that age does not matter.

---

*The data used here is imaginary and very simple. It is easier to grasp the underlying
logic and the method of carrying out the test using simple data. The method applies to any
contingency table and more realistic data is used in section 5.

[†]Although the data in a contingency table is shown as absolute numbers, the chi-square test
examines the percentage distribution pattern of the observed data compared with the expected
percentage distribution.

Table 13.2 Age of patients and length of time to specific improvement

Age in years of patients at commencement of treatment	Number of days from commencement of treatment to specific improvement			All patients	Decimal fraction*
	Under 25	25 to 49	50 and over		
Under 30	175 (135)	120 (135)	65 (90)	360	0.45
30 and under 60	105 (96)	90 (96)	61 (64)	256	0.32
60 and over	20 (69)	90 (69)	74 (46)	184	0.23
Total	300	300	200	800	1.00

*The last column contains the decimal fractions corresponding to the percentages for each age-group. These are used rather than the percentages themselves. The expected values are obtained by multiplying the sub-total for length of treatment to specific improvement (for example, 300 for under 25 days) by the decimal fraction for age-group (for example, 0.45 for under 30 years) to get the expected value of 135 corresponding to this pair of attributes.

The differences between the original data (observed values) and the values expected on the basis of no association (expected values) are therefore due to sampling error. Table 13.2 shows the original values and (in brackets) the expected values which correspond to them.

The material information in the table is the cross-tabulation of 3 categories of age by 3 categories of number of days to specific improvement. This is a (3 × 3) contingency table with 9 cells. Each cell has a unique pair of attributes, one attribute of age, one attribute of number of days to specific improvement.

Contingency tables invariably show up some differences between observed and expected values, and in this example there are clear differences suggesting that younger patients recover more quickly. Are the differences big enough to be 'real'? Or might they be due to sampling error? We explore this using the chi-square test.

We calculate the χ^2 statistic where

$$\chi^2 = \sum \frac{(o_i - e_i)^2}{e_i}$$

and o_i represents observed values, with e_i the expected value corresponding to the particular observed value.

For each of the 9 cells in the contingency table, $[(o - e)^2/e]$ is calculated, and the separate outcomes summed to give the χ^2 statistic. It is a cumulative statistic. The more cells in the contingency table, the bigger χ^2 tends to be for a given overall sample size. This is taken into account through degrees of freedom which reflect the number of ways in which the two sets of values, observed and expected, are free to vary. Not only is the total of observed and expected values the same (800), but the marginal subtotals in each age-group and in each length of treatment group are the same. Degrees of freedom are lost equal to the number of cells contained in a margin of one row and one column.* The outcome for a 3×3 contingency table is $[(3 - 1) \times (3 - 1) = 2 \times 2 = 4]$ degrees of freedom. The general statement is that for a contingency table of [r rows $\times k$ columns], the number of degrees of freedom is $[(r - 1) \times (k - 1)]$.

The calculated χ^2 statistic approximates to a theoretical chi-square distribution, a multinomial distribution. The distribution is a continuous single-tailed distribution relating frequency to values of chi-square. The total area under the curve is one. In probability terms, the fraction of area in the single tail to the right of any given value of chi-square represents the probability that this value, or a higher one, has occurred by reason of sampling error. Figure 13.1 shows the distribution of chi-square for 4 degrees of freedom.

There is a separate chi-square distribution for each number of degrees of freedom (see Appendix Table 3). We compare the calculated χ^2 statistic with the corresponding chi-square distribution having the same number of degrees of freedom, shown in the first column. Values of chi-square in each row correspond to the probability (area in the tail of the distribution) at the head of each column. As with normal curve tests, chi-square tests are conducted in probability terms. The commonly used probability level is 0.05, with extension to 0.01 and 0.001 probability levels.

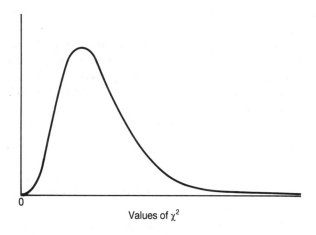

0

Values of χ^2

Figure 13.1

---

* Once the expected values for two lengths of treatment within one age-group are calculated, the third is determined by the coincidence of subtotals for both observed and expected values for that age-group. With expected values for two age-groups obtained, the remaining expected values for each category in the third age-group are again determined by the coincidence of subtotals. The loss of degrees of freedom arises from the restrictions placed on the expected values—that marginal subtotals and overall total must be the same as for the observed values.

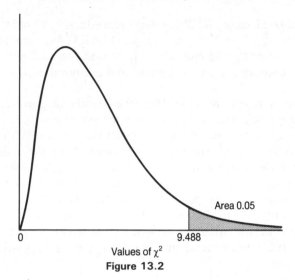

Area 0.05

0   9.488

Values of χ^2

Figure 13.2

In order to decide whether the apparent association between age and number of days to specific improvement is real or due to sampling error, we set up a Null Hypothesis of no association, that the apparent association is due to sampling error. To find the test criterion at 0.05 probability look up the table for the distribution of chi-square. Along the row for 4 degrees of freedom, the value of chi-square for 0.05 probability is 9.488 as shown in Figure 13.2.

Using the data from the contingency table, we calculate the value of χ^2.*

Table 13.3   Calculation of χ^2

(1) o values	(2) e values	(3) $o - e$	(4) $(o - e)^2$	(5) $(o - e)^2/e$
175	135	40	1600	11.851
105	96	9	81	0.844
20	69	-49	2,401	34.797
120	135	-15	225	1.667
90	96	-6	36	0.375
90	69	21	441	6.391
65	90	-25	625	6.944
61	64	-3	9	0.141
74	46	28	784	17.043
			$\sum [(o - e)^2/e] =$	80.053

---

*The calculation is not as tedious as it looks. The computation on each line must be done individually. Using a calculator this is relatively quick and the final entry (col 5) is summed in the calculator's memory. Note that the sum of the differences in col 3 is zero, as is the sum of differences in any single column or row—a useful point to remember when checking the correctness of expected values.

The calculated value, 80.053 greatly exceeds $\chi^2_{0.05}$ (9.488), and is much higher than $\chi^2_{0.01}$ (13.277) and $\chi^2_{0.001}$ (18.467). We are therefore very confident in rejecting the Null Hypothesis and concluding that there is an association between the age of patient and the number of days to specific improvement.

If we could reject the Null Hypothesis only at $p = 0.05$, we would conclude there was an association; if rejecting at $p = 0.01$, we would be more positively confident that there was an association. With the very high computed value of χ^2 we are very confident in the existence of an association between age and number of days to specific improvement. We would not reject the Null Hypothesis if the calculated value was less than the test level of $\chi^2_{0.05}$. Accepting the Null Hypothesis would require a value of χ^2 low in relation to the test level, say less than that for $p = 0.30$. We would then conclude there was no association between age and number of days to specific improvement, and that any apparent association was due to sampling error.

13.3   The Interpretation of Test Results

When rejecting the Null Hypothesis, we are positively asserting the existence of an association which cannot be attributed solely to sampling error. That does not indicate the nature of the association since the chi-square test is non-directional. We find out by looking back at the pattern of observed and expected values, and the calculation of χ^2 itself.

Looking at Table 13.2, for patients under 30 years of age more than expected improved in less than 25 days, fewer than expected in the other two improvement categories. The pattern is similar, though not so marked, for those aged 30 and under 60 years. But for those 60 years and over, far fewer than expected achieved improvement in under 25 days, with more than expected experiencing longer time to improvement.

Another pointer to where association is strong is the size of the contribution to χ^2 from the individual cells in the contingency table. Look at Table 13.3. The largest contribution to the statistic (column 5) comes from the cell associating age 60 and over with improvement in under 25 days (fewer patients than expected), followed by the cell associating age 60 and over with improvement in 50 or more days (more patients than expected), and the cell associating age under 30 with improvement in under 25 days (more patients than expected).

So there is a quite clear pattern of patients under 60 years (and more particularly those under 30 years) improving more rapidly than older patients. For patients over 60 years, relatively few improve in under 25 days. These points reinforce the initial conclusion.

13.4   The Strength of Association — The Contingency Coefficient

Where the Null Hypothesis is rejected and an association confirmed between the two sets of attributes, we may require a measure of the strength of this association. We use the contingency coefficient (C) where:

$$C = \sqrt{\frac{X^2}{X^2 + N}}$$

N being the total of all items in the contingency table (here 800).

In this example, the contingency coefficient is:

$$C = \sqrt{\frac{80.053}{80.053 + 800}} = \sqrt{\frac{80.053}{880.053}} = 0.302$$

The maximum possible value of C depends on the number of degrees of freedom. This maximum value approaches, but can never reach 1. For a 2×2 contingency table with 1 degree of freedom the maximum value of C is 0.707, and for a 3×3 contingency table with 4 degrees of freedom, the maximum value is 0.816. C can be used to compare contingency tables with the same number of degrees of freedom, but should not be used when the degrees of freedom differ.

With a value for the contingency coefficient of 0.302 against a maximum value of C of 0.816, we would look upon the association between age and number of days to specific recovery as being moderately strong.

13.5   The Formal Calculation of χ^2

The data in Table 13.4 is adapted from the GHS 1987 and shows whether or not male respondents reported limiting long standing illness by socio-economic group.

Table 13.4 Chronic sickness of males: prevalence of reported limiting long-standing illness by socio-economic group, 1987

Socio-economic group	Reporting chronic sickness	Not reporting chronic sickness	All males
Professional	123	755	878
Employers and managers	388	1,893	2,281
Intermediate and junior non-manual	348	1,699	2,047
Skilled manual and own account non-professional	877	3,506	4,383
Semi-skilled manual and personal service	427	1,429	1,856
Unskilled manual	160	457	617
Total	2,323	9,739	12,062

Source: OPCS (1989) *General Household Survey 1987*, HMSO.

To carry out a chi-square test to decide whether or not there is an association between socio-economic group and chronic sickness (reported limiting
long-standard illness), the steps are as follows:

1. Set up the Null Hypothesis that there is no association between the two
   sets of attributes, that the apparent association is due to sampling error;
2. Test the Null Hypothesis at 0.05 probability. The number of degrees of
   freedom is required $[(r - 1) \times (k - 1)]$. The value of chi-square for
   probability 0.05 and this number of degrees of freedom is the test level;
3. Calculate χ^2 where

$$\chi^2 = \sum \frac{(o - e)^2}{e}$$

4. Compare calculated χ^2 with $\chi^2_{0.05}$ and reject the Null Hypothesis if
   $\chi^2 \geq \chi^2_{0.05}$.

Following these steps:

(1) The Null Hypothesis is that there is no association between the socio-
    economic group of the respondent and whether or not chronic illness
    was reported.
(2) This is a 6×2 contingency table. There are $[(6 - 1) \times (2 - 1) = 5]$
    degrees of freedom. The critical test value of $\chi^2_{0.05}$ for 5 degrees of
    freedom is 11.070.
(3) Calculate the expected values, starting in Table 13.5 with the original
    data and adding to this. A final column has been included in the table
    showing the decimal fractions for the proportions of men in each
    socio-economic group. For example, for professional occupations, it is
    878/12,062 or 0.0728. This is recorded on the table to 4 decimal places
    (a necessary degree of accuracy), and the similar fractions calculated for
    the remaining socio-economic groups.

In practice, the easiest approach is to obtain expected values for each line
of the contingency table in turn. Taking the professional occupations, the
division $[878/12,062 = 0.0727905]$ is done on a calculator, and the result
(which will commonly be shown to 7 places of decimals, the maximum
possible for a standard pocket calculator display), stored in the calculator
memory. The decimal fraction (still on the display) is then multiplied by the
first column subtotal to give the expected value for professionals reporting
chronic sickness $[0.0727905 \times 2,323 = 169.09233$ rounded to 169].* Now
recall the decimal fraction from the memory and multiply it by the subtotal
of the second column to give the expected value for professionals not reporting chronic sickness $[0.0727905 \times 9,739 = 708.90747$, rounded to 709].

---

* If the total sample size is large as it is here, expected values recorded as whole numbers will
suffice. This eases the calculation. If in any doubt, say for samples totalling about 500 or less,
record expected values to 1 decimal place.

Table 13.5 Chronic sickness of males: prevalence of reported limiting long-standing illness by socio-economic group, 1987

Socio-economic group	Reporting chronic sickness	Not reporting chronic sickness	All males	Decimal fraction
Professional	123 (169)	755 (709)	878	0.0728
Employers and managers	388 (439)	1,893 (1,842)	2,281	0.1891
Intermediate and junior non-manual	348 (394)	1,699 (1,653)	2,047	0.1697
Skilled manual and own account non-professional	877 (844)	3,506 (3,539)	4,383	0.3634
Semi-skilled manual and personal service	427 (357)	1,429 (1,499)	1,856	0.1539
Unskilled manual	160 (119)	457 (498)	617	0.0512
Total	2,323	9,739	12,062	1.0001*

*The marginal inaccuracy in this total is not reflected in the calculations of expected values since the more accurate results from the calculator display were used.

The process is repeated for the second row. The decimal fraction for employers and managers is [2,281/12,062 = 0.1891062]. The column subtotals are multiplied by the decimal fraction to give the expected values for employers and managers reporting chronic sickness [0.1891062 × 2,323 = 439.2937, rounded to 439], and for employers and managers not reporting chronic sickness [0.1891062 × 9,739 = 1,841.7052, rounded to 1,842]. And so on, until all expected values have been computed. In Table 13.5 these are shown in brackets.

The next step is to calculate [$(o - e)^2/e$] for each cell of the contingency table as set out below. In column (1) are the observed values and in column (2) the corresponding expected values. Column (4) showing $(o - e)^2$ is not essential and can be omitted; it is included for completeness.

Table 13.6 Calculation of χ^2

(1) o	(2) e	(3) o − e	(4) $(o - e)^2$	(5) $(o - e)^2/e$
123	169	−46	2,116	12.521
388	439	−51	2,601	5.925
348	394	−46	2,116	5.371
877	844	33	1,089	1.290
427	357	70	4,900	13.725
160	119	41	1,681	14.126
755	709	46	2,116	2.984
1,893	1,842	51	2,601	1.412
1,699	1,653	46	2,116	1.280
3,506	3,539	−33	1,089	0.308
1,429	1,499	−70	4,900	3.269
457	498	−41	1,681	3.376
			$\sum [(o - e)^2/e] =$	65.587

The calculated value of χ^2 is 65.587. This is greatly in excess of $\chi^2_{0.05}$ (11.070), $\chi^2_{0.01}$ (15.086) and $\chi^2_{0.001}$ (20.515). We are therefore very confident in rejecting the Null Hypothesis and affirming that there is an association between socio-economic group and the reporting of chronic sickness.

Exploring the association by comparing observed and expected values and looking at the χ^2 calculation, we can divide the data into two broad categories. The first three socio-economic groups (professional, employers and managers, intermediate and junior non-manual) are the non-manual groups, and the second three socio-economic groups (skilled manual and own account non-professional, semi-skilled manual and personal service, unskilled manual) are the manual groups. What is notable is that for all the individual non-manual socio-economic groups, the observed values reporting chronic sickness are less than the expected. Thus for the non-manual socio-economic groups taken together, the reporting of limiting chronic sickness is less than expected. The reverse is the case for the manual socio-economic groups, where for all three the observed numbers reporting limiting chronic sickness are greater than the values expected.

Looking at the details of the χ^2 calculation, a marked difference is the fewer than expected professional men who report chronic sickness. Amongst manual workers, it is the unskilled workers and the semi-skilled manual and personal service workers in particular of whom more than expected report chronic sickness. This reinforces the general conclusion about the pattern of chronic sickness as between non-manual and manual workers.

The contingency coefficient is:

$$C = \sqrt{\frac{\chi^2}{\chi^2 + N}} = \sqrt{\frac{65.587}{65.587 + 12,062}} = \sqrt{\frac{65.587}{12,127.587}}$$

$$= \sqrt{0.005408} = 0.0736$$

This is a low value for C, and is so because the total sample size is very high in relation to the value of χ^2. The majority of the men in the sample (nearly 81%) are not reporting chronic sickness. It is from the much smaller number of those who report chronic sickness that the pattern of association appears. Although the value of C is quite low, we would still claim a marked association between socio-economic group and the reporting of chronic sickness.

We might want to make a comparison between men and women. Similar data for 12,888 women covered by the GHS 1987 generates a value of χ^2 of 140.095, much higher than that for men, and therefore indicates a stronger association between socio-economic group and chronic sickness for women compared with men. The data also shows a slightly higher percentage of women reporting chronic sickness, 22% for women compared with 19%

for men.* The value of C for the women is 0.104, which again confirms a stronger association between socio-economic group and chronic sickness for women than for men.

A Reminder

A computer will easily handle the chi-square calculation for a contingency table. At the stage of interpreting the result there is no substitute for careful consideration of the relationship between the observed and expected values and the patterns these display.

13.6 Other Chi-square Tests

The application of the chi-square test to data in contingency tables is the most common use of the test. It can be extended to any data where expected values can be computed on the basis of some hypothesis. We can test whether data have an approximately normal distribution by comparing observed frequencies with those derived from a normal distribution with the same mean, standard deviation and total frequency.[†] This can be extended to other distributions where there is an expected pattern to which we can compare observed data.

A more general example would be researching into possible changes in the severity of a particular condition. Treatment for this condition depends on whether it is classified as severe, moderate or mild. Past records show the allocation to each category as 20% severe, 45% moderate and 35% mild. Clinicians suggest that more patients are suffering from a severe form of the condition. Research conducted on 200 patients registering currently for treatment provides 50 severe cases, 65 moderate cases and 85 mild cases (observed values). We would conduct a chi-square test with expected values derived from the previous population distribution by severity of condition. These would be 20% of 200 for severe cases (40), 45% of 200 for moderate cases (90) and 25% of 200 for mild cases (50).

Table 13.7 Calculation of χ^2

Condition	o	e	$(o - e)$	$(o - e)^2$	$(o - e)^2/e$
Severe	50	40	10	100	2.500
Moderate	65	90	−25	625	6.944
Mild	85	70	15	225	3.214
				$\sum [(o - e)^2/e] =$	12.658

* This could in part be accounted for by the higher percentage of women in older age-groups, in which higher percentages of both sexes report chronic sickness.

[†] See Caulcott (1973) Chapter 7.5.

There are three pairs of observed and expected values. One degree of freedom is lost because the totals of observed and expected values are the same, leaving two [3 − 1] degrees of freedom. For two degrees of freedom the value of $\chi^2_{0.05}$ is 5.991, $\chi^2_{0.01}$ is 9.210 and $\chi^2_{0.001}$ is 13.815. We can reject the Null Hypothesis (here of 'no difference' rather than no association) at both 0.005 and 0.01 probabilities. We would confidently conclude that there is real difference between the previous pattern by severity of case and the severity of the 200 current cases in the research study. Looking at the pattern of observed and expected values, the recent research suggests an increase in both severe and mild cases, with a decline in the moderate cases.

13.7 Summary

- You have been introduced to the contingency table which sets out sample data according to two separate sets of attributes which may be numerical or categorical;
- you are aware of the flexible nature of the chi-square test in the data that can be handled, especially important that data can be non-parametric;
- the chi-square test enables you to examine the percentage distribution pattern of a series of sub-samples to decide whether or not there is an association between the two sets of attributes by which the data has been recorded in a contingency table;
- you can also use the chi-square test to examine other observed data which can be compared with a set of expected values.

Further Reading

Hoel P G and Jessen R J (1977 2nd edn) *Basic Statistics for Business and Economics* Chapter 12. New York: Wiley.
Ott L, Larson R F and Mendenhall W (1983 3rd edn) *Statistics: a Tool for the Social Sciences* Chapter 9. Boston, Mass: Duxbury Press.
Polgar S and Thomas S A (1988) *Introduction to Research in the Health Sciences* Chapter 17. Melbourne: Churchill Livingstone.

A Little Practice

1. The maternity wards of two district general hospitals had different 'preparation for childbirth schemes'. A study of patients on discharge who had participated in a scheme asked mothers to assess their satisfaction with the preparation scheme. The following were the results of the study.

Maternity patients views of 'preparation for childbirth schemes'

	Hospital A	Hospital B
Very satisfied	38	72
Fairly satisfied	83	57
Neither satisfied nor dissatisfied	42	38
Dissatisfied a little	26	44
Dissatisfied a lot	11	29
All maternity patients	200	240

Were maternity patients more satisfied with the scheme at Hospital A than Hospital B? (Test the hypothesis that there is no association between the scheme and the satisfaction expressed.)

2. Surgical patients for comparable procedures were allocated randomly to two groups of wards for postoperative care. The postoperative regimes were different in the two groups of wards. A research study recorded the length of postoperative in-patient stay for the two groups of wards.

Number of postoperative days	Group A	Group B	All patients
4 and under	46	79	125
5	42	58	100
6	36	29	65
7	20	20	40
8 and more	26	24	50
Totals	170	210	380

Does the data suggest that one regime is superior to the other regime in leading to a more prompt discharge of patients? (Test the hypothesis that there is no association between the ward regime and the number of days to discharge.)

3. A random sample of 2,500 men aged 65 years and over were asked whether they had consulted their general medical practitioner during the previous 21 days. The responses were analysed by socio-economic group.

General medical practitioner consultations in previous 21 days
Men aged 65 years and over

Socio-economic group	Had consulted	Had not consulted	All males 65 and over
Professional	42	218	260
Employers and managers	100	420	520
Intermediate and junior non-manual	105	345	450
Skilled manual and own account non-professional	161	439	600
Semi-skilled manual and personal service	102	298	400
Unskilled manual	130	140	270
Total	640	1,860	2,500

Is there an association between socio-economic group and whether or not males aged 65 and over consulted a general medical practitioner in the previous 21 days? What is the nature of the association?

4. Comparable random samples of patients suffering from a particular condition were allocated to two treatment groups. The extent of after-effects on completion of treatment was assessed. Is one form of treatment more effective than the other in controlling after-effects? (Calculate expected values to 1 place of decimals.)

	Treatment A	Treatment B	All patients
No after-effects	89	91	180
Moderate after-effects	38	42	80
Severe after-effects	23	37	60
Totals	150	170	320

14

More Data Patterns: The Analysis of Variance

14.1 The Role of Analysis of Variance

In Chapter 13, the test for differences between two sample percentages was extended to more elaborate percentage distributions of non-parametric data. We shall now extend the test for differences between two sample means to accommodate differences between the means of more than two samples.

In looking at three or more samples, we would need to consider whether the total pattern of differences between these several sample means could be attributed to sampling error, or whether there were statistically significant differences. A series of z or t-tests could be carried out between all possible pairs of sample means, but this would be clumsy, requiring multiple tests and not providing an overview of the data. A better approach is to look at the variation between the individual sample means and the overall mean (the mean of *all* the sample data) compared with the variation within the individual samples. The variation within the total sample data, and within each separate sample, is measured by the appropriate standard deviation, or its square, the variance. The variance in the total sample data can be broken down into parts; it can be analysed as variance between sample means and variance within samples. The way of doing this is called the analysis of variance or ANOVA.

The technique is much used in research based on sample data, often quite small samples, and the research design would reflect the intended analytical tool. A simple comparison between a series of samples, such as length of in-patient stay after a particular surgical procedure for patients experiencing different postoperative regimes, is looking at one experimental variable. This is known as one-way analysis of variance. The research could incorporate the effect of another variable by studying length of in-patient stay after a number of different surgical procedures. With two experimental variables, the technique is called two-way analysis of variance.

Additionally, experimental designs devised to control variation where a third variable is introduced make use of a latin square design. Research on length of in-patient stay could take account of the hospital as a further variable as well as the surgical procedure and the postoperative regime.

ANOVA is based on a number of assumptions. Firstly, that the samples are random, the common prerequisite for statistical inference. Secondly, that each sample comes from a population which is itself a normal distribution. Thirdly, that all the populations from which the samples are drawn have the same standard deviation.

Much data approximates sufficiently to the normal distribution for ANOVA to be used. If nothing is known about the population itself we look to the sample data as guide. With a reasonable 'bunching' of values centrally in the sample data and relatively few extreme values, the second condition is met. Provided the standard deviations of the separate samples do not greatly differ, that the majority of values fall within an approximately similar range, the third condition is met.

Stressing these points may appear to add complications, but they are part of the framework in which ANOVA operates. If the second and third conditions clearly are not met, ANOVA is not an appropriate technique.

14.2   One-way Analysis of Variance

A research study covers three groups of patients being treated for the same skin condition, each group experiencing a different treatment. The three groups show different outcomes in terms of the mean number of days to specific improvement.

The question that arises is 'Are the differences in the mean number of days to specific improvement due to the different treatments? Or are the differences the result of sampling error? In commonsense terms, if the variation *within* each of the samples is small (for each treatment, the individual numbers of days to specific improvement are all fairly close to the mean for that sample group), the different treatments are providing consistent results. But if the differences between mean days to specific improvements are large as *between* samples (between treatments) then there could be differences between sample means not attributable to sampling error. This would lead to the conclusion that some treatment(s) were more or less effective than others.

As with normal curve tests, we set up a Null Hypothesis that there is no difference between the sample means, that the samples all come from the same population ($\mu_1 = \mu_2 = \mu_3$). We need a suitable criterion for deciding whether or not to reject the Null Hypothesis and shall make use of a theoretical distribution known as the F distribution.

F is a ratio between two independent estimates of the variance in the population from which the samples are derived. The first estimate of the variance is based on the variance between the means of the separate samples and the mean of all the sample data taken together. The second estimate is obtained as a mean of the variance of the separate samples. The first estimate measures the variation between the sample means, the second measures the variation within the samples. If the first estimate is large compared with the second estimate then it is possible that there are real differences between the sample means, not due to sampling error. We can compute the F ratio and test it against the properties of the theoretical F distribution using an appropriate probability level.

Table 14.1 shows the number of days to specific improvement for the three groups each of eight patients given different treatments for a skin condition.

Table 14.1   Number of days to specific improvement

	Treatment A	Treatment B	Treatment C
	36	41	44
	38	44	48
	44	48	39
	37	39	45
	40	44	50
	46	47	41
	37	43	46
	42	46	47
Sample mean	40 days	44 days	45 days
Sample standard deviation	3.43 days	2.83 days	3.39 days
Sample variance	11.75 days	8 days	11.5 days

The data is for k ($= 3$) samples each of size n ($= 8$), so the overall sample size, N is [$k \times n = 24$] patients. The mean of all samples taken together ($\bar{x}$) is 43 days. Figure 14.1 shows the values in the three samples, their individual means, and the mean of all the data. This gives an impression of the variations within and between the samples.

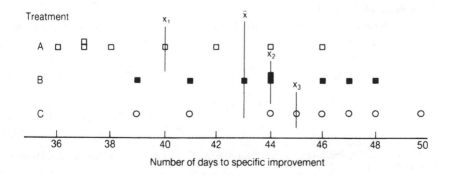

Figure 14.1

The first estimate of the variance is based on the variance between the means of each of the three samples (x_1, x_2, and x_3) and their overall mean ($\bar{x}$). Using s_b^2 to indicate the variance between the sample means:*

$$s_b^2 = \frac{n[(x_1 - \bar{x})^2 + (x_2 - \bar{x})^2 + (x_3 - \bar{x})^2]}{k - 1}$$

where n is the common sample size and k the number of samples, with [$k - 1$] the number of degrees of freedom for s_b^2. One degree of freedom is lost through the calculation of the overall mean.

This can be expressed in general terms for k samples, each size n, where x_i is the mean for the representative individual sample:

$$s_b^2 = \frac{n[\sum x_i^2 - \{(\sum x_i)^2/k\}]}{k - 1}$$

Inserting the sample data:

$$s_b^2 = \frac{8 \times [40^2 + 44^2 + 45^2 - (40 + 44 + 45)^2/3]}{2}$$

$$= \frac{8 \times [1{,}600 + 1{,}936 + 2{,}025 - (129)^2/3}{2}$$

$$= \frac{8 \times [5{,}561 - 16{,}641/3]}{2}$$

$$= \frac{8 \times [5{,}561 - 5{,}547]}{2} = \frac{8 \times 14}{2} = 56$$

The second estimate of the variance is the mean of the variances of the individual samples. The general expression is:†

$$s_w^2 = \frac{\sum s_i^2}{k}$$

where s_i^2 is the variance of the representative sample and k is the number of samples of equal size.

Using the sample variances from Table 14.1 above, the second estimate of the variance s_w^2 is:

$$s_w^2 = \frac{s_1^2 + s_2^2 + s_3^2}{k}$$

$$= \frac{11.75 + 8 + 11.5}{3} = \frac{31.25}{3} = 10.42$$

---

* The subscript 'b' indicates that s_b^2 is the estimate of variance based on differences between the sample means.

† The subscript 'w' indicates that s_w^2 is the estimate of population variance based on variance within the samples.

This second estimate is derived from three samples, each of eight patients. The number of degrees of freedom is equal to the total sample size (24 patients) less one degree of freedom for each separate sample mean (3) calculated. Degrees of freedom are $[N - k]$, here 21 degrees of freedom.

The two independent estimates of the population variance are s_b^2 ($= 56$) and s_w^2 ($= 10.42$). The first estimate (variation between the sample means) is clearly much bigger than the second estimate (variance within the samples), but is the first *sufficiently* larger to indicate that the samples are different, are not from the same population?

We compute the ratio:

$$F = \frac{\text{Variation between sample means}}{\text{Variation within samples}} = \frac{s_b^2}{s_w^2} = \frac{56}{10.42} = 5.37$$

In order to decide whether to reject the Null Hypothesis calculated F is compared with the theoretical distribution of F. The distribution depends on the two figures for degrees of freedom. There are separate distributions of F for each combination of degrees of freedom for numerator and denominator respectively.

As a test criterion we use the conventional 0.05 probability, with 0.01 probability for more stringent testing or for expanding on the test results. The F distribution is an asymmetrical distribution with a single tail, similar to the chi-square distribution. The probability of a particular value of F (or a higher one) occuring is the proportion of total area in the tail of the F distribution.

Tables of F are set out with degrees of freedom for numerator and denominator respectively for a particular probability level. In Appendix Table 4 there are two tables of F, for 0.05 and 0.01 probability.* For any particular example, the F value for the appropriate degrees of freedom is looked up in the table for the chosen test criterion. If the calculated F ratio is greater than or equal to this value, the Null Hypothesis is rejected.

In this example, there are 2 degrees of freedom in the numerator, 21 in the denominator. Looking up the table of values of $F_{0.05}$, the test value of F is 3.47, considerably less than the calculated F (5.37). For the table for $F_{0.01}$ the F value is 5.78. The probability of the F ratio having occurred by chance is less than 0.05, and not much in excess of 0.01. This is shown in Figure 14.2. We are confident in rejecting the Null Hypothesis.

There is therefore a real difference between the two measures of the variance, and the samples cannot be viewed as coming from the same population. The different treatments have different outcomes to an extent

---

*More extensive tables of F for additional probability levels can be found in volumes of statistical tables such as Pearson and Hartley (1966 3rd edn).

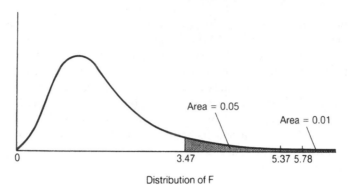

Distribution of F

Figure 14.2

greater than can be accounted for by sampling error. Treatment A shows notably fewer days to specific improvement compared with Treatments B and C.

Note. Equal sample sizes leads to advantages in the reliability of the F statistic and to minimal risks of making a Type II error. ANOVA can be carried out for unequal samples and the formulae are:

$$s_b^2 = \frac{\sum x_i^2 n_i - [(\sum x_i n_i)^2/N]}{k - 1}$$

and

$$s_w^2 = \frac{\sum (n_i - 1)s_i^2}{N - k}$$

where x_i is the mean of the representative sample with size n_i and variance s_i^2. There are k samples and total sample size is N where $N = \sum n_i$.

14.3   The Formal Steps

The procedure for the analysis of variance is similar to that already established for a chi-square test.

1. The Null Hypothesis is set up, that there is no difference between the sample means, and that any observed difference is due to sampling error.
2. A probability level is selected for testing the Null Hypothesis, commonly 0.05.
3. The F ratio is calculated.
4. The degrees of freedom for numerator and denominator are determined and $F_{0.05}$ for these degrees of freedom obtained. Calculated F is compared to this test level. If $F \geq F_{0.05}$, conclusions are also drawn against $F_{0.01}$.

5. If the Null Hypothesis is rejected, then the pattern of differences between the sample means cannot be attributed to sampling error, but is due to other causes. The direction and nature of the underlying differences is determined from the research data, not from the test result.

14.4   Conclusion and Interpretation

What conclusion would we draw from this example? That the samples must be looked upon as coming from different populations. The different treatments cannot be viewed as having similar outcomes, differing only to an extent that can be accounted for by sampling error. Treatment A shows notably fewer days to specific improvement. Treatments B and C have very similar results.*

ANOVA is most useful when data are available from a number of samples. It is important to ensure that distribution between the sample groups, in this example the different treatments, is made by a random process. Additionally patients could be matched and then distributed randomly between the separate samples (see Chapter 9.4). It is important to ensure that no other variable (age of patient, length of time the patient has suffered from the condition, previous treatment) could have led to different results between the samples.

Analysis of variance has analogies with the chi-square test. Both deal with more complex situations which involve a number of samples. In both, the test result indicates a pattern not attributable to sampling error, but does not indicate the direction of the association (chi-square) or the nature of the pattern (analysis of variance). We must look at the data and what that tells us in order to draw conclusions.

14.5   Two-way Analysis of Variance

A second variable, severity of condition when treatment commenced, could be incorporated into the research study of patients receiving different treatments for a particular skin condition. Suppose there are four classifications of severity, which with three treatments gives the following two-way classification. The table shows the distribution of twelve patients, three for each severity of condition, distributed randomly between the three treatments.

---

* A significance test conducted on the difference between the means of samples B and C would not lead to rejecting the Null Hypothesis. The calculation of t produces a very low value, 0.64; the probability of the difference between the means of samples B and C occurring through sampling error is between 0.5 and 0.6, slightly in excess of one half. There is no evidence that treatment B is superior to treatment C.

Table 14.2 Patients suffering from a skin condition: Severity of condition at commencement and treatment given

Severity of condition	Treatment A	Treatment B	Treatment C
Mild	1	2	3
Moderate	4	5	6
Severe	7	8	9
Very severe	10	11	12

The research design allows for one observation, one patient, in each cell. The study can be replicated, providing several patients in each cell. A replicated study has the advantage of increasing overall sample size, with an improved likelihood of firm conclusions, and the possibility of taking into account any interaction between variables. With more than one observation for each combination of severity of condition and treatment, replication enables variability between patients to be taken into account.

Two way analysis of variance provides two Null Hypotheses to be tested:

1. that there is no difference in the lapse of time to specific improvement between patients with difference severities of condition; and
2. that there is no difference in the lapse of time to specific improvement between patients receiving different treatments.

The separate Null Hypotheses are tested against $F_{0.05}$ for the appropriate degrees of freedom. Conclusions are drawn in the same way as for one-way analysis of variance.

Computation is complex and is best done by computer so seek appropriate software. For those who wish to pursue an understanding of the computation, see Further Reading.

14.6   Experimental Designs — The Latin Square

Suppose we are interested in the effect of different postoperative regimes in reducing the length of in-patient stay after surgical procedures. A research project taking place at four hospitals is studying four different postoperative regimes following four different surgical procedures. In total there are 64 different combinations possible from the three variables $[4 \times 4 \times 4 = 64]$. In practice these can be reduced to the much more manageable number of 16 different experimental groups as shown in Table 14.3. The four different postoperative regimes are A, B, C and D.

Each surgical procedure appears four times, associated with one of each of the four postoperative regimes, and with each of the four hospitals. Research at each hospital covers all four surgical procedures and all four

Table 14.3 Research design for effectiveness of postoperative regimes

Surgical procedure	Hospital			
	H_1	H_2	H_3	H_4
1	A	B	C	D
2	D	A	B	C
3	C	D	A	B
4	B	C	D	A

postoperative regimes. The net effects is to balance out the role of the three variables and to produce a more compact research project.

The latin square design allows three Null Hypotheses to be tested:

1. that there is no difference in the length of in-patient stay for patients who have had different surgical procedures;
2. that there is no difference in the length of in-patient stay for patients who have experienced different postoperative regimes; and
3. that there is no difference in length of in-patient stay for patients in different hospitals.

The computer output will include the three values of F (or the means of obtaining them) which can be compared with $F_{0.05}$. Conclusions can be drawn in the same way as for one-way analysis of variance.

As for two-way ANOVA, computations are best done by computer. The output will include the three values of F required for testing the three Null Hypotheses. For those who wish to look further into the computational method, see Further Reading.

14.7   Summary

- You have now extended comparison between sample means to more than two samples;
- in one-way analysis of variance you are testing whether the overall variation between the individual sample means is more than can be accounted for (in probability terms) by sampling error;
- two-way analysis of variance extends the research design to include a second variable, and leads to testing two Null Hypotheses;
- you can extend the research design further to accommodate a third variable and the testing of three Null Hypotheses;
- after rejecting any Null Hypothesis you must examine carefully the pattern of the differences between the samples in order to draw conclusions;
- the calculations for ANOVA are complex and should be done by computer.

Further Reading

For a more mathematical discussion, including extensions to more than two variables:

Freund J E (1979 5th edn) *Modern Elementary Statistics* Chapter 16. London: Prentice/Hall.

Hoel P G and Jessen R J (1977 2nd edn) *Basic Statistics for Business and Economics* Chapter 13. New York: Wiley.

Ott L, Larson R F and Mendenhall W (1983 3rd edn) *Statistics: a Tool for the Social Sciences* Chapter 12. Boston, Mass: Duxbury Press.

Walpole R E (1982 3rd edn) *Introduction to Statistics* Chapter 12. New York: Collier: Macmillan.

A Little Practice

The advice to readers is to use computers for ANOVA computations. Following are two simple examples for those who wish to try one-way analysis of variance using a calculator.

1. Research in a particular ward using three different analgesics provided the following results for the length of time the analgesic relieved pain for thirty patients in the immediate postoperative period.

Number of hours pain relieved

Analgesic A	Analgesic B	Analgesic C
3	2.5	3.5
2.5	4	2.5
4	4.5	4
2	2.5	4.5
5	3.5	5
3.5	2	3.5
3	3	4
4	2.5	3
4.5	3.5	3.5
3.5	3	4.5

Use one-way ANOVA to test whether there is any difference between the three analgesics in their effectiveness in relieving postoperative pain.

2. Twenty-four patients suffering from a particular skin condition of approximately the same severity were randomly divided into three groups. Each group was given a different treatment, and the number of courses of treatment required to achieve a specific improvement was noted.

Number of courses of treatment required

Treatment A	Treatment B	Treatment C
3	3	7
1	5	4
4	6	6
2	4	4
3	4	7
5	8	5
3	7	8
7	3	7

Do the research results suggest there is any difference between the treatments in their effectiveness?

Part IV

Analysis

15

Regression

15.1 The Regression Line

The statistical analysis described in this chapter involves two (or more) variables consisting of interval data. We seek a means of measuring the change in one variable (y, the dependent variable) consequent upon changes in another variable (x, the independent variable). A relationship established between the dependent and the independent variables can be used to *predict* a mean value of the dependent variable corresponding to a given value of the independent variable. Chapter 16 deals with the strength of this association.

Research could look at the relationship between length in days of a course of treatment (independent variable) and outcome in number of days to specific improvement (dependent variable), at the age of patients at the onset of a condition and the days to measured improvement, or at the age on entry to training of student nurses and the percentage in each age-group passing the final examination at the first attempt.

The relationship we shall set up between the dependent and independent variables is linear, a straight line. It is known as a regression line, because the line represents the values to which those of the dependent variable (for given value of the independent variable) are expected to regress. Mathematically, it is the 'line of best fit'; the regression line passes through the mean of all values and fits as closely as possible to the data.*

The general equation for a straight line is

$$y = a + bx$$

In the present context a and b are referred to as regression coefficients; a is the intercept on the y-axis when $x = 0$, and b is the slope or gradient of the line. Usefully, b can be thought of as measuring the change in y when x changes by one. Either a or b can be negative. When b is positive,

---

*If pairs of values of the two variables are plotted graphically, the regression line passes through the mean of the array of points, and the sum of the squared distances of the points from the line is a minimum.

y increases when x increases; this is referred to as a positive relationship. When b is negative, y will decrease as x increases and vice versa; this is a negative relationship.

For sets of paired values of any two variables, it is possible to calculate two regression lines. With two variables, A and B, we can calculate a regression line in which variable A is treated as independent and variable B as dependent. If we treat variable B as independent and variable A as dependent, we obtain a different regression line. The first line would represent mean values of the dependent variable B corresponding to values of the independent variable A. From this we could predict a mean value of B for any given value of A. The second line does the reverse; it represents the mean values of the dependent variable A for given values of the independent variable B, enabling us to predict mean A for given values of B.

We have to take a positive decision about which is the independent and which the dependent variable. In the great majority of actual situations, there is a clear independent variable, and a clear dependent variable. There would therefore be only one regression line that we would wish to obtain. Think carefully about dependence and independence; if in doubt ask the question 'which variable can lead to changes in the other?'

15.2 The Scatter Diagram

A useful preliminary is to plot the data graphically on a scatter diagram. The values of the independent variable, x, are plotted on the horizontal axis, the x-axis. The values of the dependent variable, y, are plotted on the vertical axis, the y-axis.* This gives a general impression of the relationship between x and y, whether it is fairly close, or whether the paired values (x, y) are very scattered. If well scattered, this would suggest a limited relationship between x and y. The scatter diagram also shows whether high or low values of both variables go together, or whether high values of one variable go with low values of the other and vice versa.

15.3 An Example

Suppose we have data for twenty patients on the length of time between commencing a course of treatment for a particular skin condition and the achievement of a specific improvement. The results suggest improvement is more speedy the earlier treatment is commenced after the condition has been diagnosed. We have the following data for the patients.

---

* Naming the independent variable 'x' and the dependent variable 'y', plotting values of x on the horizontal axis and of y on the vertical axis, follows conventional algebraic rules.

Table 15.1 Lapse of time from diagnosis to commencement of treatment and length of treatment to specific improvement: patients suffering from a particular skin condition

Patient	Weeks to treatment	No. of days to improvement	Patient	Weeks to treatment	No. of days to improvement
1	2	12	11	7	27
2	3	18	12	8	44
3	3	24	13	9	31
4	4	14	14	9	42
5	4	26	15	10	57
6	4	32	16	11	43
7	5	40	17	11	35
8	6	22	18	11	59
9	7	34	19	12	43
10	7	23	20	12	51

The data are shown on the scatter diagram, Figure 15.1.

Both the data and the scatter diagram demonstrate that there is a relationship between the two variables, lapse of time from diagnosis to treatment and length of treatment. The relationship appears to be moderately close, and it is positive; longer lapses of time from diagnosis to commencement of treatment are associated with longer periods of treatment to specific improvement.

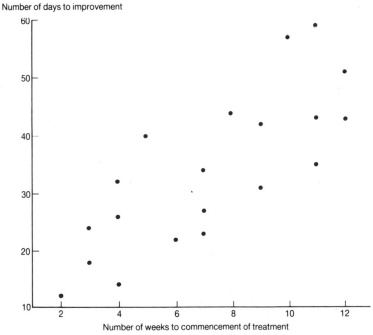

Figure 15.1

Regression coefficients are derived from the following expressions, b being calculated first and then used to obtain a:

$$b = \frac{n \sum x_i y_i - \sum x_i \sum y_i}{n \sum x_i^2 - (\sum x_i)^2} \quad \text{and} \quad a = \frac{\sum y_i - b \sum x_i}{n}$$

where x_i and y_i represent a pair of values of x and y, and n is the number of pairs of values. The calculation of the summations set out in Table 15.2 is similar in form to that for the mean and standard deviation.

Table 15.2 Weeks to treatment and number of days to improvement

Patient	Weeks to treatment (x)	No. of days to improvement (y)	xy	x^2
1	2	12	24	4
2	3	18	54	9
3	3	24	72	9
4	4	14	56	16
5	4	26	104	16
6	4	32	128	16
7	5	40	200	25
8	6	22	132	36
9	7	34	238	49
10	7	23	161	49
11	7	27	189	49
12	8	44	352	64
13	9	31	279	81
14	9	42	378	81
15	10	57	570	100
16	11	43	473	121
17	11	35	385	121
18	11	59	649	121
19	12	43	516	144
20	12	51	612	144
Totals	$\sum x = 145$	$\sum y = 677$	$\sum xy = 5{,}572$	$\sum x^2 = 1{,}255$

We now have

$$b = \frac{n \sum xy - \sum x \sum y}{n \sum x^2 - (\sum x)^2} = \frac{20 \times 5{,}572 - 145 \times 677}{20 \times 1{,}255 - (145)^2}$$

$$= \frac{111{,}440 - 98{,}165}{25{,}100 - 21{,}025} = \frac{13{,}275}{4{,}075} = 3.258$$

and

$$a = \frac{\sum y - b \sum x}{n} = \frac{677 - 3.258 \times 145}{20}$$

$$= \frac{677 - 472.41}{20} = 10.23$$

The regression equation is $y = 10.23 + 3.258x$.

15.4 Predicting From the Regression Equation

Having derived the equation of a regression line, values of x can be inserted to obtain corresponding values of y. Suppose we wish to predict the mean length of time to specific improvement for patients for whom the lapse of time between diagnosis and the commencement of treatment was 10 weeks. Inserting $x = 10$:

$$y = 10.23 + 3.258 \times 10 = 10.23 + 32.58 = 42.81$$

For patients for whom the lapse of time between diagnosis and commencement of treatment was 10 weeks the mean time to improvement is 43 days.

15.5 Points on Interpretation

We have already noted the matter of positive and negative relationships, depending on the sign or direction of b. As x increases by one, y will change by b, either an increase (b is positive) or a decrease (b is negative). The scatter diagram shows whether the relationship appears to be fairly close—or otherwise. Plotting the regression line on the scatter diagram gives a further visual impression. Select two reasonably well spaced values of x and obtain the corresponding values of y. Plot the two pairs of values of x and y, and join them to form a straight line. This is shown in Figure 15.2.*

If the relationship between the two variables is not very close, the values of y will be well scattered round the regression line and any predicted values of y (points on the regression line for given values of x) are unlikely to be very meaningful. On the other hand, if the points lie close to the line, predicted values of y will be much more reliable. A formal measure of the closeness with which the points lie to the line is pursued in Chapter 16.

The regression line is computed from a specific set of values. If we added more pairs of values of x and y (or subtracted some), the regression line would be different. The line depends on the precise information used to obtain it. Each pair of values of x and y has equal weight in the computation.

---

*An accurate line is plotted if the two points are well apart, so use the extreme values of x in the data ($x = 2$, $x = 12$).

$$x = 2, \qquad y = 10.23 + 3.258 \times 2 = 10.23 + 6.516 = 16.75$$

$$x = 12, \qquad y = 10.23 + 3.258 \times 12 = 10.23 + 39.096 = 49.33$$

These pairs of values (2, 16.8) and (12, 49.3) are used in Figure 15.2 to plot the regression line.

Number of days to improvement

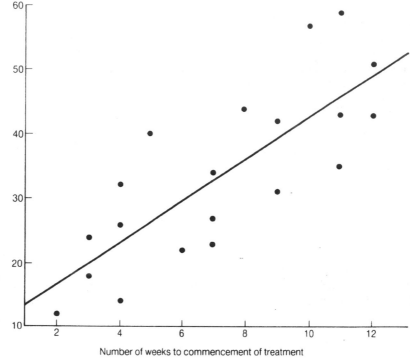

Number of weeks to commencement of treatment

Figure 15.2

When predicting from the regression line, we are reasonably safe in predicting within the range of values to which the data relate (interpolation), but are not so safe in predicting outside this range of values (extrapolation). It does not follow that the relationship established by the regression line will be the same for values outside the range of the data from which the line is derived. The relationship may very well be different, and indeed there are many circumstances in which extrapolating to any substantial extent would be wrong. In addition, in positive relationships, it may not be possible for values to rise continuously; in negative relationships, declining values of y with rising values of x may lead to impossible negative values of y.

We have considered a *linear* relationship between two variables. It gives a straightforward relationship, easy to understand and to use. What if the underlying relationship is not linear? A straight line may still be a good and useful approximation of the relationship between the variables over the range of values to which data relate. Where the underlying relationship is not linear, or is unlikely to extend in linear form outside the data, we must be very cautious in extrapolating from it.

For a non-linear relationship between x and y there may be other algebraic equations which are a better expression of the relationship between the variables. These can be pursued but fitting an elaborate curve to data may give no serious advantage and could itself be misleading.

Finally, the ability to obtain a regression line (and that the relationship appears close) does not necessarily indicate a meaningful relationship. Never lose sight of any limitations in the data and the reasonableness of the relationship established. That we can obtain a linear relationship between independent and dependent variables does not prove the relationship is causal. Whilst a good regression relationship supports causality, causality itself depends on factors outside statistical analysis.

15.6   Regression Over Time

The regression line technique can be used to fit a line to time series data. This is a rather special line and there are additional limitations to its value and use.

The following list of data sets out annual neonatal death rates for the UK (deaths of infants under four weeks of age per thousand live births) for years from 1961 to 1988.

Table 15.3   Neonatal death rates (UK): 1961–1988

Year	Rate	Year	Rate
1961	15.8	1978	8.8
1966	13.2	1979	8.3
1969	12.3	1980	7.7
1970	12.5	1981	6.7
1971	12.0	1982	6.4
1972	11.7	1983	5.9
1973	11.4	1984	5.7
1974	11.3	1985	5.4
1975	10.9	1986	5.3
1976	9.9	1987	5.0
1977	9.5	1988	4.9

Source: OPCS (1975, 1981, 1986, 1990) *Population Trends 1, 26, 46, 62* HMSO.

Neonatal mortality rates fell steadily over this period which is emphasised in Figure 15.3.

Note that chronological time is shown on the x-axis and the neonatal death rate on the y-axis. Time is always the independent variable. Change takes place on account of the passage of time and what is subsumed therein. To calculate a regression line from these data recode time (the nominal years from 1961 onwards) on a convenient scale. Equal intervals of time

Neonatal death rates

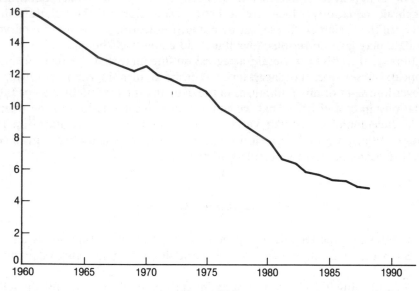

Figure 15.3

are represented by equal intervals on the scale, an increase of 1 represents one year. Recode 1961 as 1, 1966 as 6, 1969 as 9, 1970 as 10 etc. to 1988 which will be 28. The basic calculations are shown in Table 15.4.

Substituting into the formulae for the regression coefficients:

$$b = \frac{n \sum xy - \sum x \sum y}{n \sum x^2 - (\sum x)^2} = \frac{22 \times 2,962 - 377 \times 200.6}{22 \times 7,547 - 377^2}$$

$$= \frac{65,164 - 75,626.2}{166,034 - 142,129} = \frac{-10,462.2}{23,905} = -0.438$$

$$a = \frac{\sum y - b \sum x}{n} = \frac{200.6 + 0.438 \times 377\,*}{22}$$

$$= \frac{200.6 + 165.126}{22} = \frac{365.726}{22} = 16.62$$

The regression equation shows a negative relationship:

$$y = 16.62 - 0.438x \qquad (x = 1 \text{ in } 1961)$$

---

 * As b is negative, change the direction of the immediately preceding sign. This itself is minus so the sign becomes a plus. The same occurs in the equation of the regression line; the negative value of b changes the preceding plus sign to a minus.

Table 15.4 Neonatal death rates (UK): 1961–1988

Year	Rate (y)	x	xy	x^2
1961	15.8	1	15.8	1
1966	13.2	6	79.2	36
1969	12.3	9	110.7	81
1970	12.5	10	125	100
1971	12.0	11	132	121
1972	11.7	12	140.4	144
1973	11.4	13	148.2	169
1974	11.3	14	158.2	196
1975	10.9	15	163.5	225
1976	9.9	16	158.4	256
1977	9.5	17	161.5	289
1978	8.8	18	158.4	324
1979	8.3	19	157.7	361
1980	7.7	20	154	400
1981	6.7	21	140.7	441
1982	6.4	22	140.8	484
1983	5.9	23	135.7	529
1984	5.7	24	136.8	576
1985	5.4	25	135	625
1986	5.3	26	137.8	676
1987	5.0	27	135	729
1988	4.9	28	137.2	784
	$\sum y = 200.6$	$\sum x = 377$	$\sum xy = 2,962$	$\sum x^2 = 7,547$

What can we tell from the regression line? The regression coefficient b, here -0.438, gives the mean annual *decline* in the neonatal death rate between 1961 and 1988. Recollect that all values of neonatal deaths play an equal part in the calculation of the regression line. What happened in 1961 or for that matter 1970 or 1980 is of much less importance in predicting the future than what happened in 1988, 1987 and other more recent years. Further, neonatal deaths could not go on declining at the same rate, as that implies a negative value by 1998!

Looking at the information in more detail, is the pattern the same over the whole period (27 years)? Suppose the data are taken in three equal periods of 9 years (1961–1970, 1970–1979, and 1979–1988).* We can construct three separate regression equations:

$$
\begin{aligned}
1961–1970 \qquad & y = 15.97 - 0.388x \\
1970–1979 \qquad & y = 17.32 - 0.461x \\
1979–1988 \qquad & y = 14.64 - 0.362x
\end{aligned}
\left. \begin{aligned} \\ \\ \\ \end{aligned} \right\} x = 1 \text{ in } 1961
$$

The three separate lines are shown in Figure 15.4.

---

*Annual data relates to the mid-point of the year (30 June/1 July), so the time period is from mid-1961 to mid-1988, 27 years.

Neonatal death rates

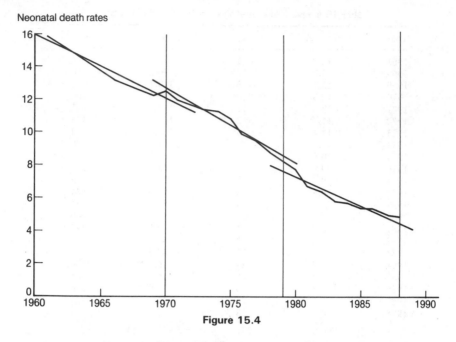

Figure 15.4

The mean decline in the first period of nine years was 0.39 per annum; there was a rather sharper decline over the next nine years, 0.46 per annum, but this reduced over the last period of nine years to 0.36 per annum— an interesting pattern. When time-series data are declining, the *rate* of decline itself is likely to fall. The value of y (neonatal death rate) must always be positive; the lower the existing level of the neonatal death rate, the more modest the scope for further reductions. The most recent rate of decline is less than for earlier years which confirms the lesser scope for future reductions. It is the pattern of recent years that will most clearly indicate possible directions in the immediate future.

Can we use time-series regression lines for prediction? Crystal ball gazing is a bit tricky. Predictions can only be valid if the pattern of time immediately past is likely to be followed in the future. Validity can only hold for the immediate future, not for the distant future. We might consider using the last of the three regression lines (1979–1988) to predict neonatal rates for, say, 1990. Replacing x with 30 in the regression equation:

$$y = 14.64 - 0.362 \times 30 = 14.64 - 10.86 = 3.78 \text{ (rounded to 3.8)}.$$

Setting this against the last years of the data (5.0 in 1987, 4.9 in 1988), a predicted neonatal death rate of 3.8 in 1990 looks decidedly uncertain. Predicting for 1992 gives a value of 3.1 which is even more uncertain. The past rate of decline in the neonatal death rate is most unlikely to be continued into the future; the rate of decline itself appears to be falling.

A similar problem arises when data over time are rising (a positive relationship) as when they are falling. There may be an upper limit as with the percentage of children immunised against diphtheria which cannot exceed 100%. The higher the percentage immunised, the less the scope for further improvement. We would expect a decline in the *rate* at which the percentage immunised rose. Early improvements may be relatively easy to achieve; later ones much more difficult. Data which are rising over time may by nature show reduced future improvement. Favourable circumstances are unlikely to continue indefintely.

The regression line records what has happened in the past. It may provide a measure against which to judge the future. Extreme caution is necessary when predicting that the past will continue into future, even the very immediate future.

15.7   Multiple Regression

We can establish a relationship between a dependent variable, y, and several independent variables, x_1, x_2, x_3, etc. This would lead to a multiple regression equation:

$$y = a + b_1 x_1 + h_2 x_2 + b_3 x_3 \text{ etc.}$$

In the example in section 3 above about the relationship between lapse of time to commencement of treatment and number of days to specific improvement, younger patients might appear to recover more quickly. Age could be taken into account as a second independent variable. A large number of patients would be required for such an exercise to be realistic—a group of 20 is inadequate. Suitable computer software would be required to carry out the more complicated calculations. Taking into account a second independent variable could be highly informative in establishing what influenced the rapidity of improvement. See also Chapter 16.7 and 16.8.

15.8   Summary

- You have been introduced to an important area of data analysis, linear regression, concerning the relationship between two variables, one of which is independent and the other dependent;
- you have learnt to draw a scatter diagram, to obtain a simple regression line to express the relationship between two sets of variable values, and to use your regression line for prediction;
- you have included the special technique of deriving a regression line from time-series data;

- you are aware of the limitations of the technique you are using;
- you understand that extensions to the regression relationship are possible using more than one independent variable.

Note. A proper understanding of regression relationships requires also an understanding of correlation which is covered in the following chapter. Further Reading and examples for the two chapters are therefore included at the end of Chapter 16.

16

Correlation

16.1 The Strength of Relationships

In Chapter 15 we explored the relationship between variables through the regression line, and now extend this to consider the *strength* of the regression relationship.

We can always establish a linear regression relationship between two variables, but for that relationship to be helpful it must be reasonably strong. It has to be meaningful to say that changes in the independent variable will lead to changes in the dependent variable. The more closely the regression line fits to the data, the more important the independent variable is in determining values of the dependent variable.

Data from the natural and physical sciences may demonstrate very close relationships; data from the medical and social sciences in which the role of individual variability is strong, may demonstrate much less close relationships. The correlation coefficient measures the closeness of a relationship between two variables. The most commonly used correlation coefficient is based on the numerical values of parametric data. The rank correlation coefficient which uses ordinal data is covered in section 6. Reference to a correlation coefficient should be taken as reference to the common form based on numerical values which is also known as the product moment correlation coefficient.

16.2 The Product Moment Correlation Coefficient

In Chapter 14 we made use of the variance in analysing relationships, and shall make use of it again in the context of correlation. The variance in the values of y (the dependent variable) can be broken down into explained and unexplained variance. Explained variance is that accounted for by the regression relationship between the two variables; unexplained variance is the variance not accounted for by the regression relationship.

In Figure 16.1 point M $(\bar{x}, \bar{y})$ represents the mean of values of x and y respectively; point A (x_i, y_i) is any pair of values from the data. Point B is the point on the regression line corresponding to value x_i. We will call

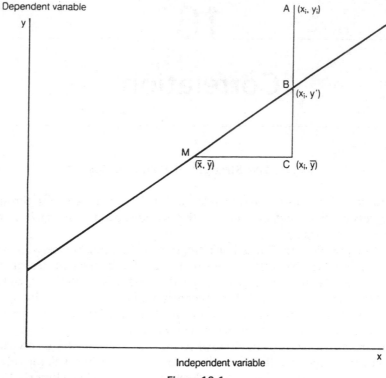

Figure 16.1

this point (x_i, y'). Point C represents x_i plotted against the mean of the dependent variable y, so C is the point $(x_i, \bar{y})$. AC $(y_i - \bar{y})$ is a measure related to total variance in the values of y; BC $(y' - \bar{y})$ is a measure related to the explained variance; and AB $(y_i - y')$ is a measure related to the unexplained variance. So the total variance between values of y (values of the dependent variable) and $\bar{y}$ (the mean of all the y values) is broken down into explained variance (that which is accounted for by the regression relationship) and unexplained variance (that which is represented as the scatter of y values round the regression line).

The correlation coefficient (r) is defined as:

$$r = \sqrt{\frac{\text{explained variance}}{\text{total variance}}} = \sqrt{\frac{\Sigma\,(y' - \bar{y})^2}{\Sigma\,(y_i - \bar{y})^2}}$$

The closer the points of the scatter diagram lie to the regression line and the closer the relationship between x and y, the larger the explained variance in relation to total variance, and the higher the value of r. The sign of r, its direction, can be positive or negative and is the same as that of the regression coefficient b. If the regression relationship is negative, the calculation of r will engender a negative value. The value of r lies between -1 and $+1$, but what is important is its *magnitude* between zero and ± 1. A very low value of $|r|$, close to zero, indicates no relationship between x and y; the higher the arithmetic value of $|r|$, the closer the relationship between the two variables. A very high value of r, say ± 0.9 or above, indicates a very strong relationship between the two variables.

16.3 The Calculation of the Correlation Coefficient

The expression for obtaining r is:

$$r = \frac{n \sum x_i y_i - \sum x_i \sum y_i}{\sqrt{[n \sum x_i^2 - (\sum x_i)^2][n \sum y_i^2 - (\sum y_i)^2]}}$$

which requires a basic calculation similar to that for the regression line, but with the addition of the summation $\sum y^2$. Note that it is easy to obtain r, the correlation coefficient, at the same time as the regression line. We use the data on patients suffering from a particular skin condition from Chapter 15.

Table 16.1 Lapse of time from diagnosis to commencement of treatment and length of treatment to specific improvement: patients suffering from a particular skin condition

Patient	Weeks to treatment (x)	No. of days to improvement (y)	xy	x^2	y^2
1	2	12	24	4	144
2	3	18	54	9	324
3	3	24	72	9	576
4	4	14	56	16	196
5	4	26	104	16	676
6	4	32	128	16	1,024
7	5	40	200	25	1,600
8	6	22	132	36	484
9	7	34	238	49	1,156
10	7	23	161	49	529
11	7	27	189	49	729
12	8	44	352	64	1,936
13	9	31	279	81	961
14	9	42	378	81	1,764
15	10	57	570	100	3,249
16	11	43	473	121	1,849
17	11	35	386	121	1,225
18	11	59	649	121	3,481
19	12	43	516	144	1,849
20	12	51	612	144	2,601
Totals	$\sum x = 145$	$\sum y = 677$	$\sum xy = 5,572$	$\sum x^2 = 1,255$	$\sum y^2 = 26,353$

Substituting in the formula:

$$r = \frac{n \sum xy - \sum x \sum y}{\sqrt{[n \sum x^2 - (\sum x)^2][n \sum y^2 - (\sum y)^2]}}$$

$$r = \frac{20 \times 5,572 - 145 \times 677}{\sqrt{[20 \times 1,255 - 145^2][20 \times 26,353 - 677^2]}}$$

$$= \frac{111,440 - 98,165}{\sqrt{[25,100 - 21,025][527,060 - 458,329]}} = \frac{13,275}{\sqrt{4,075 \times 68,731}}$$

$$= \frac{13,275}{16,736} = 0.793$$

This is a fairly high value of r, and shows a reasonably strong association between the two variables.

16.4   Points on Interpretation

The calculation of r does not require one variable to be independent and the other to be dependent. The algebraic formula is symmetrical and would result in an identical value for r if x was replaced by y and y by x. Whereas there are two regression lines (the regression of y on x, and the regression of x on y, with the first named variable as the dependent variable), there is only one correlation coefficient measuring the strength of the relationship between the two variables.

Since r varies between 0 and ± 1, with *magnitude* indicating strength of association, we can devise a rough scale* to assist in interpreting values of r.

0.9 and above—very strong association

0.8   —fairly strong association

0.6–0.7   —moderate association

0.4–0.5   —weak association

0.2–0.3   —very weak association

0.1 and under—no association

Remember that the sign indicates the *direction* of association. The positive sign means high values of x go with high values of y, and low with low; the negative sign that high values of x go with low values of y, and vice versa. This is exactly the same as with the regression coefficient, b.

---

*The scale refers to the magnitude of the *arithmetic* values of r, irrespective of the direction sign. So a value of r of $+0.75$ represents a moderately strong positive relationship between the variables, a value of -0.75 representing an equally strong negative relationship.

We can conduct a significance test on r. If there is no correlation between the two variables, r will be zero. The Null Hypothesis would be that there is no difference between the calculated value of r and its hypothesised value of zero, and that the observed difference is due to sampling error. We use the expression

$$z \text{ (or } t) = \frac{r}{se_r}$$

where the standard error of r (se_r) when $r = 0$, is $1/\sqrt{(n - 2)}$.*

The degrees of freedom for this expression are $(n - 2)$, and t is used rather than z if $(n - 2)$ is 30 or less. In this example the degrees of freedom are 18:

$$t = \frac{r}{se_r}$$

$$se_r = 1/\sqrt{(20 - 2)} = 1/\sqrt{18} = 1/4.243 = 0.236$$

Therefore

$$t = \frac{0.793}{0.236} = 3.360$$

Looking up the table of t-values for 18 degrees of freedom, $t_{0.05} = 2.093$, $t_{0.01} = 2.861$ and $t_{0.001} = 3.883$. The Null Hypothesis is rejected at 0.05 and 0.01 probability (but not at 0.001 probability). We would therefore be very confident in asserting that there was a reasonably strong association between the lapse of time from diagnosis to the commencement of treatment, and the time to specific improvement. The time lapse between diagnosis and commencement of treatment is associated with a longer time from commencement of treatment to specific improvement.

Another way of looking at r is to do so through the coefficient of determination, $r^2 \times 100$. This is the percentage of the variation in the dependent variable which is attributable to the independent variable. In this example, the coefficient of determination is 63%. Over three fifths of the variation in the time to specific improvement is accounted for by the lapse of time between diagnosis and the commencement of treatment.

———————

Very important note. The correlation coefficient, r, is strictly a measure of association. It does not imply causation. High values of r do not of themselves prove that changes in x cause changes in y to occur. Spurious correlations are common. If seeking to establish causation in the relationship

———————

*The general expression for se_r is:

$$se_r = \frac{1 - r^2}{n - 2}$$

and can be used to construct confidence limits for any calculated value of r.

between two variables we require good grounds, for reasons other than their statistical association, to be confident a relationship does exist. Additionally, changes in x (the independent variable) must precede changes in y (the dependent variable). We must be confident that the relationship is between x and y; that there is no other variable that could be responsible for the pattern of changes in both x and y.

Finally, do not forget that the correlation coefficient relates to the strength of the *linear* relationship between the two variables. Relationships are not necessarily linear; nonetheless the correlation coefficient may be a reasonable guide to the strength of the association between the variables, particularly over a limited range of values.

16.5 Time-Series Data and Correlation

In Chapter 15.6 we discussed reasons for exercising caution over using time-series data for prediction. As measured by the magnitude of r, the regression line fits very closely to time-series data. This is because there is only one value of y for each time-point and in practical terms the change that is possible between successive time-points is limited. The value of $|r|$ can be very high even although the scatter diagram indicates that the regression line will not be reliable for prediction. In the time-series example on neonatal death rates, the value of r is -0.9886. Our initial conclusion that the regression line derived from this data could not be used for prediction is not changed by the high value of $|r|$.

16.6 The Rank Correlation Coefficient

If data can be placed in rank order, a correlation coefficient can be calculated from the rankings. This is valuable in that the measure accommodates ordinal non-parametric data, for example ranked preferences, satisfaction with information or treatment given, assessments of severity of a condition.

The formula for the rank correlation coefficient (r') is

$$r' = 1 - \frac{6 \sum d_i^2}{n(n^2 - 1)}$$

The values of x and y are separately ranked, d_i is the difference between the ranks of the paired values (x_i, y_i), and n the number of pairs of values.*

---

*This formula is a rearrangement of the formula for the product moment correlation coefficient, incorporating the mathematical effect of variables x and y each consisting of the numbers 1 to n. The sum of the consecutive numbers 1 to n and the sum of their squares can be expressed in terms of n. A final rearrangement produces the rank correlation coefficient formula.

When handling the data there are two points to note. It must be treated consistently—either high values ranked from one, or low values ranked from one, but both variables treated the same. If values are identical, they must have the same rank order. To achieve this, if two equal values relate to ranks 4 and 5, each is given the midpoint rank 4.5. The next rank to be allocated will be rank 6. If three values are equal, covering ranks 4, 5 and 6, they will take the midpoint rank of 5, and the next rank to be allocated will be 7. As an example the data from Table 16.1 is used to calculate r'.

Table 16.2 Lapse of time from diagnosis to commencement of treatment and length of treatment to specific improvement: patients suffering from a particular skin condition

Patient	Weeks to treatment (x)	No. of days to improvement (y)	Rank x	Rank y	Difference between ranks (d)	Difference squared (d^2)
1	2	12	1	1	0	0
2	3	18	2.5	3	0.5	0.25
3	3	24	2.5	6	3.5	12.25
4	4	14	5	2	3	9
5	4	26	5	7	2	4
6	4	32	5	10	5	25
7	5	40	7	13	6	36
8	6	22	8	4	4	16
9	7	34	10	11	1	1
10	7	23	10	5	5	25
11	7	27	10	8	2	4
12	8	44	12	17	5	25
13	9	31	13.5	9	4.5	20.25
14	9	42	13.5	14	0.5	0.25
15	10	57	15	19	4	16
16	11	43	17	15.5	1.5	2.25
17	11	35	17	12	5	25
18	11	59	17	20	3	9
19	12	43	19.5	15.5	4	16
20	12	51	19.5	18	1.5	2.25
Total						$\sum d^2 = 248.5$

The rank correlation coefficient is:

$$r' = 1 - \frac{6 \sum d^2}{n(n^2 - 1)}$$

$$= 1 - \frac{6 \times 248.5}{20(20^2 - 1)} = 1 - \frac{1,491}{20 \times 399}$$

$$= 1 - \frac{1,491}{7,980} = 1 - 0.186 = 0.813$$

The value for r' is slightly higher than that obtained for r (0.793), but the two values do not greatly differ.

Why should we use r' rather the r? What are the advantages of the rank correlation coefficient?

1. Data may be non-parametric but consist of characteristics which can be put in rank order thereby enabling a rank correlation coefficient to be obtained.
2. Data which take on numerical values may include extreme and well scattered values. A product moment correlation coefficient could be a distorted measure and a rank correlation coefficient a better indicator of the association between the variables. Alternatively, deficiencies in the numerical data could make a rank correlation coefficient preferable.
3. The relationship between the variables may not be linear. If the relationship is curvilinear, the rank correlation coefficient could be a better estimate of the strength of the association between the two variables. The more the data deviate from the linear relationship, the more appropriate would be the rank correlation coefficient.

A final point; if the data have numerical values, use the product moment correlation coefficient, unless there are good reasons for doing otherwise.

16.7 Multiple Correlation

We can obtain a multiple correlation coefficient to study the closeness of fit of the data to the configuration represented by a multiple regression equation.* The suggestion for the example in Chapter 15.7 that age should be taken into account as a second independent variable in addition to lapse of time from diagnosis to commencement of treatment would lead to calculating a multiple correlation coefficient for the three variables. If we calculated three simple correlation coefficients between successive pairs of the three variables, we might find some correlation not only between age and days of treatment to specific improvement, but also between age and lapse of time from diagnosis to commencement of treatment. This would be useful information in itself. It would emphasise the *relative* importance of age and lapse of time from diagnosis to treatment in determining the outcome of treatment. The *direction* of the correlation between age and the lapse of time to commencement of treatment would indicate whether older patients might be being handicapped by later commencement of treatment (a positive correlation).

---

*With two independent variables, the multiple regression equation represents a three dimensional configuration—a plane. With more than two independent variables, the multi-dimensional geometrical configuration is one we cannot even envisage.

The multiple correlation coefficient takes into account the simple correlations betwen pairs of the three variables. It measures the overall strength of association between them, and the closeness of fit of the data to the geometrical plane represented by the regression equation.

16.8 Partial Correlation

This is an alternative way of looking at the relationship in which an additional variable is involved. It measures the correlation between two variables, controlling for the effect of a second independent variable. We could have examined the data on the patients with a skin condition in this way, controlling for the age of the patients (thereby eliminating any correlation attributable to this variable) and obtaining a partial correlation coefficient between the lapse of time from diagnosis to the commencement of treatment and the time to specific improvement.

The introduction of an additional variable with either multiple or partial correlation offers a greater range of possibilities for both association and causation, and can be explored through the Further Reading.

––––––––––

The benefit of computers is very considerable in the area covered by this and the preceding chapter. Any statistical software package will include regression and correlation, including standard errors and the coefficient of determination. For multiple regression and multiple and partial correlation, computer packages are essential tools. It is important to understand this area of statistics; but make use of the computer.

Many scientific calculators are programmed to handle linear regression and correlation. They have the disadvantage of not providing a record of data inserted and are only practical for small quantities of data. Beware the risks of error when entering values.

16.9 Summary

- You have extended your analysis of the relationship between variables to correlation, to a means of measuring the strength of the association between two variables;
- you are able to calculate the product moment correlation coefficient between two variables where both take on numerical values;
- you can conduct a significance test, and examine the strength of the association through the coefficient of determination;
- you can calculate the rank correlation coefficient where data is non-parametric and can be ranked, or where a rank correlation coefficient would otherwise be appropriate;

- you are aware of the possibility of extending correlation analysis to more than two variables;
- you know of the importance of correlation in establishing a statistical association which can support but cannot prove the presence of a causal relationship.

Further Reading

Blalock H M (1972 2nd edn) *Social Statistics* Chapter 17–19. Tokyo: McGraw-Hill Kogakusha.

Freund J E and Williams F J (1970 2nd edn) *Modern Business Statistics* Chapters 13 and 14. London: Pitman.

Hoel P G and Jessen R J (1977 2nd edn) *Basic Statistics for Business and Economics* Chapters 9–11. New York: Wiley.

Ott L, Larson R F and Mendenhall W (1983) *Statistics: a Tool for the Social Sciences* Chapter 11. Boston, Mass: Duxbury Press.

Reid N G and Boore R P (1987) *Research Methods and Statistics in Health Care* Chapter 6. London: Edward Arnold.

A Little Practice

1. The out-patient clinic administrator is anxious to avoid wastage of staff time because booked patients do not attend clinics and wishes to introduce a policy of deliberately overbooking. Data on booked patients and numbers attending a particular clinic were collected for 16 out-patient sessions.

Clinic session	Number of patients booked	Number attending
1	40	37
2	42	39
3	40	34
4	38	36
5	39	38
6	41	40
7	37	35
8	37	33
9	38	36
10	38	37
11	40	40
12	41	39

13	42	38
14	36	34
15	38	37
16	37	37

The target size of clinic session is 40 patients. The out-patient manager wants to know (a) the mean expected attendance if 40 patients are booked, and (b) the number of patients who should be booked to achieve a mean attendance of 40 patients. (Obtain a regression line which enables attendances to be predicted from number of patients booked. Using the regression line (a) predict the mean number of attendances if 40 patients are booked ($x = 40$), and (b) determine the number of bookings that should be made to obtain a predicted mean value of 40 for attendances ($y = 40$).)

2. In a particular hospital district a programme to reduce the wastage of student nurses in training has resulted in the following wastage rates over fifteen consecutive intakes of students.

Intake	Wastage rate (percentage of intake)
1	16
2	18
3	24
4	20
5	15
6	16
7	21
8	20
9	18
10	20
11	17
12	14
13	18
14	17
15	15

(a) Present the above data graphically.
(b) From the data obtain the equation of the regression line from which the mean percentage wastage rate could be predicted for future intakes.
(c) What has been the average change in wastage rates between intakes? [Look at the regression coefficient, b.]
(d) Predict the mean wastage rates for intakes 17 and 20. Do you think these levels can be achieved?

3. The marks for twelve student nurses in a written examination and in a practical examination are compared.

| | Examination marks (out of 50) | |
Student	Written	Practical
1	19	32
2	24	33
3	32	38
4	38	40
5	23	30
6	42	41
7	29	37
8	44	39
9	36	39
10	28	33
11	39	38
12	36	36

Calculate the coefficient of correlation between the marks of the student nurses in the two examinations. How would you interpret this as a measure of association?

4. Two nurse assessors jointly interview applicants for student nurse training and then make individual decisions about the suitability of each applicant for nurse training by awarding a score between 1 and 20. Their scores for 15 applicants are as follows.

Applicant	Assessor A	Assessor B
1	7	8
2	14	9
3	10	7
4	16	12
5	13	8
6	18	11
7	17	13
8	9	7
9	8	9
10	20	16
11	12	10
12	18	15
13	19	19
14	19	17
15	15	10

(a) Draw a scatter diagram for the data.
(b) Calculate (i) the product moment correlation coefficient and (ii) the rank correlation coefficient.
(c) Do you think there is a reasonable degree of agreement between the two assessors? Which measure is more appropriate?

17

Postscript

No book on statistics can include everything that each reader might wish to find in it. For the author, selectivity is essential. In Part I, I have tried to deal with aspects of basic data which in my view receive less attention in texts than they deserve, and than many readers, hesitant about handling numerical material, would wish. Descriptive statistics in Part II are discussed and presented with the aim of giving the user a good understanding both of the measures and of the way in which data is handled logically. In approaching both Part I and Part II, we require to develop a crude sense of the quantitative, what orders of magnitude are right, what makes sense.

In dealing with inferential statistics in Part III, I have concentrated on the more robust statistical tests which give strong guidance on differences and patterns arising from sample data, and that are therefore likely to lead to firm conclusions. These are not restricted to parametric tests; chi-square is a powerful non-parametric test. Sample percentages arise from non-parametric data, whether nominal or ordinal, since they are simple head counting exercises of the sample units that do and that do not possess a particular characteristic. Tests for differences involving sample percentages are therefore valuable for non-parametric data. The rank correlation coefficient (Part IV) is a non-parametric measure of association applicable to ordinal data.

There are additional tests for non-parametric sample data, not covered in this book, which should only be used when the more powerful tests are not applicable. The main non-parametric tests are discussed in Walpole (1982) Chapter 13. A more comprehensive review of non-parametric measures is to be found in Siegel and Castellan (1988).

Finally, Part IV on analysis is an introduction to relationships between variables, an area which readers may wish to pursue further, both in extending simple correlation and regression to incorporate additional variables, and in more complex analysis, such as Factor Analysis. This is an area for computers.

An important aim throughout this book has been to provide an adequate explanation of basic principles underlying statistical techniques. Be sure the techniques you use are appropriate; be sure the conclusions are justified.

Do not attempt to extract more information than is really contained in the data, or than can be inferred through statistical measures.

A last reminder—never forget the importance of commonsense, never lose awareness of the underlying relationship between statistical results and the nature of the data to which these apply. Statistical techniques do not offer a magic wand to solve all problems; they are part of the tools that are available to us in analysing data and in drawing sensible and valuable conclusions from it. Be self-critical and questioning in all you do.

Appendix

Statistical Tables

1. Normal curve areas
2. Distribution of t
3. Distribution of chi-square
4. Distribution of F

Statistics for Nurses

Appendix: Statistical Tables

Table 1   Normal curve areas

The table entry corresponds to the shaded area for the particular value of z.

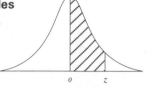

z	0.00	0.01	0.02	0.03	0.04	0.05	0.06	0.07	0.08	0.09
0.0	0.0000	0.0040	0.0080	0.0120	0.0160	0.0199	0.0239	0.0279	0.0319	0.0359
0.1	0.0398	0.0438	0.0478	0.0517	0.0557	0.0596	0.0636	0.0675	0.0714	0.0753
0.2	0.0793	0.0832	0.0871	0.0910	0.0948	0.0987	0.1026	0.1064	0.1103	0.1141
0.3	0.1179	0.1217	0.1255	0.1293	0.1331	0.1368	0.1406	0.1443	0.1480	0.1517
0.4	0.1554	0.1591	0.1628	0.1664	0.1700	0.1736	0.1772	0.1808	0.1844	0.1879
0.5	0.1915	0.1950	0.1985	0.2019	0.2054	0.2088	0.2123	0.2157	0.2190	0.2224
0.6	0.2257	0.2291	0.2324	0.2357	0.2389	0.2422	0.2454	0.2486	0.2517	0.2549
0.7	0.2580	0.2611	0.2642	0.2673	0.2704	0.2734	0.2764	0.2794	0.2823	0.2852
0.8	0.2881	0.2910	0.2939	0.2967	0.2995	0.3023	0.3051	0.3078	0.3106	0.3133
0.9	0.3159	0.3186	0.3212	0.3238	0.3264	0.3289	0.3315	0.3340	0.3365	0.3389
1.0	0.3413	0.3438	0.3461	0.3485	0.3508	0.3531	0.3554	0.3577	0.3599	0.3621
1.1	0.3643	0.3665	0.3686	0.3708	0.3729	0.3749	0.3770	0.3790	0.3810	0.3830
1.2	0.3849	0.3869	0.3888	0.3907	0.3925	0.3944	0.3962	0.3980	0.3997	0.4015
1.3	0.4032	0.4049	0.4066	0.4082	0.4099	0.4115	0.4131	0.4147	0.4162	0.4177
1.4	0.4192	0.4207	0.4222	0.4236	0.4251	0.4265	0.4279	0.4292	0.4306	0.4319
1.5	0.4332	0.4345	0.4357	0.4370	0.4382	0.4394	0.4406	0.4418	0.4429	0.4441
1.6	0.4452	0.4463	0.4474	0.4484	0.4495	0.4505	0.4515	0.4525	0.4535	0.4545
1.7	0.4554	0.4564	0.4573	0.4582	0.4591	0.4599	0.4608	0.4616	0.4625	0.4633
1.8	0.4641	0.4649	0.4656	0.4664	0.4671	0.4678	0.4686	0.4693	0.4699	0.4706
1.9	0.4713	0.4719	0.4726	0.4732	0.4738	0.4744	0.4750	0.4756	0.4761	0.4767
2.0	0.4772	0.4778	0.4783	0.4788	0.4793	0.4798	0.4803	0.4808	0.4812	0.4817
2.1	0.4821	0.4826	0.4830	0.4834	0.4838	0.4842	0.4846	0.4850	0.4854	0.4857
2.2	0.4861	0.4864	0.4868	0.4871	0.4875	0.4878	0.4881	0.4884	0.4887	0.4890
2.3	0.4893	0.4896	0.4898	0.4901	0.4904	0.4906	0.4909	0.4911	0.4913	0.4916
2.4	0.4918	0.4920	0.4922	0.4925	0.4927	0.4929	0.4931	0.4932	0.4934	0.4936
2.5	0.4938	0.4940	0.4941	0.4943	0.4945	0.4946	0.4948	0.4949	0.4951	0.4952
2.6	0.4953	0.4955	0.4956	0.4957	0.4959	0.4960	0.4961	0.4962	0.4963	0.4964
2.7	0.4965	0.4966	0.4967	0.4968	0.4969	0.4970	0.4971	0.4972	0.4973	0.4974
2.8	0.4974	0.4975	0.4976	0.4977	0.4977	0.4978	0.4979	0.4979	0.4980	0.4981
2.9	0.4981	0.4982	0.4982	0.4983	0.4984	0.4984	0.4985	0.4985	0.4986	0.4986
3.0	0.49865	0.49869	0.49874	0.49878	0.49882	0.49886	0.49889	0.49893	0.49896	0.49900
3.1	0.49903	0.49906	0.49910	0.49913	0.49916	0.49918	0.49921	0.49924	0.49926	0.49929
3.2	0.4993129									
3.3	0.4995166									
3.4	0.4996631									
3.5	0.4997674									
3.6	0.4998409									
3.7	0.4998922									
3.8	0.4999277									
3.9	0.4999519									
4.0	0.4999683									
4.5	0.4999966									
5.0	0.4999997133									
z	0.00	0.01	0.02	0.03	0.04	0.05	0.06	0.07	0.08	0.09

This table is adapted from Table 1 of E S Pearson and H O Hartley (eds), *Biometrika Tables for Statisticians* Vol 1, third edition (1966) by permission of the *Biometrika* trustees.

Table 2 Distribution of t

Probability refers to the proportion of total area
(shaded) in the two tails of the t distribution for
computed values of t at the appropriate degrees
of freedom. This applies to two-tailed tests; the
probability is *halved* for one-tailed tests.

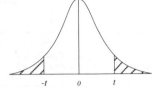

Degrees of freedom	Probability												
	0.9	0.8	0.7	0.6	0.5	0.4	0.3	0.2	0.1	0.05	0.02	0.01	0.001
1	0.158	0.325	0.510	0.727	1.000	1.376	1.963	3.078	6.314	12.706	31.821	63.657	636.619
2	0.142	0.289	0.445	0.617	0.816	1.061	1.386	1.886	2.920	4.303	6.965	9.925	31.598
3	0.137	0.277	0.424	0.584	0.765	0.978	1.250	1.638	2.353	3.182	4.541	5.841	12.924
4	0.134	0.271	0.414	0.569	0.741	0.941	1.190	1.533	2.132	2.776	3.747	4.604	8.610
5	0.132	0.267	0.408	0.559	0.727	0.920	1.156	1.476	2.015	2.571	3.365	4.032	6.869
6	0.131	0.265	0.404	0.553	0.718	0.906	1.134	1.440	1.943	2.447	3.143	3.707	5.959
7	0.130	0.263	0.402	0.549	0.711	0.896	1.119	1.415	1.895	2.365	2.998	3.499	5.408
8	0.130	0.262	0.399	0.546	0.706	0.889	1.108	1.397	1.860	2.306	2.896	3.355	5.041
9	0.129	0.261	0.398	0.543	0.703	0.883	1.100	1.383	1.833	2.262	2.821	3.250	4.781
10	0.129	0.260	0.397	0.542	0.700	0.879	1.093	1.372	1.812	2.228	2.764	3.169	4.587
11	0.129	0.260	0.396	0.540	0.697	0.876	1.088	1.363	1.796	2.201	2.718	3.106	4.437
12	0.128	0.259	0.395	0.539	0.695	0.873	1.083	1.356	1.782	2.179	2.681	3.055	4.318
13	0.128	0.259	0.394	0.538	0.694	0.870	1.079	1.350	1.771	2.160	2.650	3.012	4.221
14	0.128	0.258	0.393	0.537	0.692	0.868	1.076	1.345	1.761	2.145	2.624	2.977	4.140
15	0.128	0.258	0.393	0.536	0.691	0.866	1.074	1.341	1.753	2.131	2.602	2.947	4.076
16	0.128	0.258	0.392	0.535	0.690	0.865	1.071	1.337	1.746	2.120	1.583	2.921	4.015
17	0.128	0.257	0.392	0.534	0.689	0.863	1.069	1.333	1.740	2.110	2.567	2.898	3.965
18	0.127	0.257	0.392	0.534	0.688	0.862	1.067	1.330	1.734	2.101	2.552	2.878	3.922
19	0.127	0.257	0.391	0.533	0.688	0.861	1.066	1.328	1.729	2.093	2.539	2.861	3.883
20	0.127	0.257	0.391	0.533	0.687	0.860	1.064	1.325	1.725	2.086	2.528	2.845	3.850
21	0.127	0.257	0.391	0.532	0.686	0.859	1.063	1.323	1.721	2.080	2.518	2.831	3.819
22	0.127	0.256	0.390	0.532	0.686	0.858	1.061	1.321	1.717	2.074	2.508	2.819	3.792
23	0.127	0.256	0.390	0.532	0.685	0.858	1.060	1.319	1.714	2.069	2.500	2.807	3.767
24	0.127	0.256	0.390	0.531	0.685	0.857	1.059	1.318	1.711	2.064	2.492	2.797	3.745
25	0.127	0.256	0.390	0.531	0.684	0.856	1.058	1.316	1.708	2.060	2.485	2.787	3.725
26	0.127	0.256	0.390	0.531	0.684	0.856	1.058	1.315	1.706	2.056	2.479	2.779	3.707
27	0.127	0.256	0.389	0.531	0.684	0.855	1.057	1.314	1.703	2.052	2.473	2.771	3.690
28	0.127	0.256	0.389	0.530	0.683	0.855	1.056	1.313	1.701	2.048	2.467	2.763	3.674
29	0.127	0.256	0.389	0.530	0.683	0.854	1.055	1.311	1.699	2.045	2.462	2.756	3.659
30	0.127	0.256	0.389	0.530	0.683	0.854	1.055	1.310	1.697	2.042	2.457	2.750	3.646
40	0.126	0.255	0.388	0.529	0.681	0.851	1.050	1.303	1.684	2.021	2.423	2.704	3.551
60	0.126	0.254	0.387	0.527	0.679	0.848	1.046	1.296	1.671	2.000	2.390	2.660	3.460
120	0.126	0.254	0.386	0.526	0.677	0.845	1.041	1.289	1.658	1.980	2.358	2.617	3.373
∞	0.126	0.253	0.385	0.524	0.674	0.842	1.036	1.282	1.645	1.960	2.326	2.576	3.291
Degrees of freedom	Probability												
	0.9	0.8	0.7	0.6	0.5	0.4	0.3	0.2	0.1	0.05	0.02	0.01	0.001

Table 2 is taken from Table III of Fisher and Yates': *Statistical Tables for Biological, Agricultural and Medical Research* published by Longman Group UK Ltd, London (previously published by Oliver and Boyd Ltd, Edinburgh) and by permission of the authors and publishers.

Table 3   Distribution of chi-square

Probability refers to the proportion of total area
(shaded) in the single tail of the chi-square
distribution for computed values of χ^2
at the appropriate degrees of freedom.

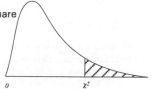

Degrees of freedom	Probability											
	0.95	0.90	0.80	0.70	0.50	0.30	0.20	0.10	0.05	0.02	0.01	0.001
1	0.00393	0.0158	0.0642	0.148	0.455	1.074	1.642	2.706	3.841	5.412	6.635	10.827
2	0.103	0.211	0.446	0.713	1.386	2.408	3.219	4.605	5.991	7.824	9.210	13.815
3	0.352	0.584	1.005	1.424	2.366	3.665	4.642	6.251	7.815	9.837	11.345	16.266
4	0.711	1.064	1.649	2.195	3.357	4.878	5.989	7.779	9.488	11.668	13.277	18.467
5	1.145	1.610	2.343	3.000	4.351	6.064	7.289	9.236	11.070	13.388	15.086	20.515
6	1.635	2.204	3.070	3.828	5.348	7.231	8.558	10.645	12.592	15.033	16.812	22.457
7	2.167	2.833	3.822	4.671	6.346	8.383	9.803	12.017	14.067	16.622	18.475	24.322
8	2.733	3.490	4.594	5.527	7.344	9.524	11.030	13.362	15.507	18.168	20.090	26.125
9	3.325	4.168	5.380	6.393	8.343	10.656	12.242	14.684	16.919	19.679	21.666	27.877
10	3.940	4.865	6.179	7.267	9.342	11.781	13.442	15.987	18.307	21.161	23.209	29.588
11	4.575	5.578	6.989	8.148	10.341	12.899	14.631	17.275	19.675	22.618	24.725	31.264
12	5.226	6.304	7.807	9.034	11.340	14.011	15.812	18.549	21.026	24.054	26.217	32.909
13	5.892	7.042	8.634	9.926	12.340	15.119	16.985	19.812	22.362	25.472	27.688	34.528
14	6.571	7.790	9.467	10.821	13.339	16.222	18.151	21.064	23.685	26.873	29.141	36.123
15	7.261	8.547	10.307	11.721	14.339	17.322	19.311	22.307	24.996	28.259	30.578	37.697
16	7.962	9.312	11.152	12.624	15.338	18.418	20.465	23.542	26.296	29.633	32.000	39.252
17	8.672	10.085	12.002	13.531	16.338	19.511	21.615	24.769	27.587	30.995	33.409	40.790
18	9.390	10.865	12.857	14.440	17.338	20.601	22.760	25.989	28.869	32.346	34.805	42.312
19	10.117	11.651	13.716	15.352	18.338	21.689	23.900	27.204	30.144	33.687	36.191	43.820
20	10.851	12.443	14.578	16.266	19.337	22.775	25.038	28.412	31.410	35.020	37.566	45.315
21	11.591	13.240	15.445	17.182	20.337	23.858	26.171	29.615	32.671	36.343	38.932	46.797
22	12.338	14.041	16.314	18.101	21.337	24.939	27.301	30.813	33.924	37.659	40.289	48.268
23	13.091	14.848	17.187	19.021	22.337	26.018	28.429	32.007	35.172	38.968	41.638	49.728
24	13.848	15.659	18.062	19.943	23.337	27.096	29.553	33.196	36.415	40.270	42.980	51.179
25	14.611	16.473	18.940	20.867	24.337	28.172	30.675	34.382	37.652	41.566	44.314	52.620
26	15.379	17.292	19.820	21.792	25.336	29.246	31.795	35.563	38.885	42.856	45.642	54.052
27	16.151	18.114	20.703	22.719	26.336	30.319	32.912	36.741	40.113	44.140	46.963	55.476
28	16.928	18.939	21.588	23.647	27.336	31.391	34.027	37.916	41.337	45.419	48.278	56.893
29	17.708	19.768	22.475	24.577	28.336	32.461	35.139	39.087	42.557	46.693	49.588	58.302
30	18.493	20.599	23.364	25.508	29.336	33.530	36.250	40.256	43.773	47.962	50.892	59.703
Degrees of freedom	Probability											
	0.95	0.90	0.80	0.70	0.50	0.30	0.20	0.10	0.05	0.02	0.01	0.001

Table 3 is taken from Table IV of Fisher and Yates': *Statistical Tables for Biological, Agricultural and Medical Research* published by Longman Group UK Ltd, London (previously published by Oliver and Boyd Ltd, Edinburgh) and by permission of the authors and publishers.

Table 4(a)   Distribution of F

The table entry is the critical value of F at 0.05 probability corresponding to the appropriate degrees of freedom for numerator (v_1) and denominator (v_2).

v_2 \ v_1	1	2	3	4	5	6	7	8	9	10	12	15	20	24	30	40	60	120	∞
1	161.4	199.5	215.7	224.6	230.2	234.0	236.8	238.9	240.5	241.9	243.9	245.9	248.0	249.1	250.1	251.1	252.2	253.3	254.3
2	18.51	19.00	19.16	19.25	19.30	19.33	19.35	19.37	19.38	19.40	19.41	19.43	19.45	19.45	19.46	19.47	19.48	19.49	19.50
3	10.13	9.55	9.28	9.12	9.01	8.94	8.89	8.85	8.81	8.79	8.74	8.70	8.66	8.64	8.62	8.59	8.57	8.55	8.53
4	7.71	6.94	6.59	6.39	6.26	6.16	6.09	6.04	6.00	5.96	5.91	5.86	5.80	5.77	5.75	5.72	5.69	5.66	5.63
5	6.61	5.79	5.41	5.19	5.05	4.95	4.88	4.82	4.77	4.74	4.68	4.62	4.56	4.53	4.50	4.46	4.43	4.40	4.36
6	5.99	5.14	4.76	4.53	4.39	4.28	4.21	4.15	4.10	4.06	4.00	3.94	3.87	3.84	3.81	3.77	3.74	3.70	3.67
7	5.59	4.74	4.35	4.12	3.97	3.87	3.79	3.73	3.68	3.64	3.57	3.51	3.44	3.41	3.38	3.34	3.30	3.27	3.23
8	5.32	4.46	4.07	3.84	3.69	3.58	3.50	3.44	3.39	3.35	3.28	3.22	3.15	3.12	3.08	3.04	3.01	2.97	2.93
9	5.12	4.26	3.86	3.63	3.48	3.37	3.29	3.23	3.18	3.14	3.07	3.01	2.94	2.90	2.86	2.83	2.79	2.75	2.71
10	4.96	4.10	3.71	3.48	3.33	3.22	3.14	3.07	3.02	2.98	2.91	2.85	2.77	2.74	2.70	2.66	2.62	2.58	2.54
11	4.84	3.98	3.59	3.36	3.20	3.09	3.01	2.95	2.90	2.85	2.79	2.72	2.65	2.61	2.57	2.53	2.49	2.45	2.40
12	4.75	3.89	3.49	3.26	3.11	3.00	2.91	2.85	2.80	2.75	2.69	2.62	2.54	2.51	2.47	2.43	2.38	2.34	2.30
13	4.67	3.81	3.41	3.18	3.03	2.92	2.83	2.77	2.71	2.67	2.60	2.53	2.46	2.42	2.38	2.34	2.30	2.25	2.21
14	4.60	3.74	3.34	3.11	2.96	2.85	2.76	2.70	2.65	2.60	2.53	2.46	2.39	2.35	2.31	2.27	2.22	2.18	2.13
15	4.54	3.68	3.29	3.06	2.90	2.79	2.71	2.64	2.59	2.54	2.48	2.40	2.33	2.29	2.25	2.20	2.16	2.11	2.07
16	4.49	3.63	3.24	3.01	2.85	2.74	2.66	2.55	2.54	2.49	2.42	2.35	2.28	2.24	2.19	2.15	2.11	2.06	2.01
17	4.45	3.59	3.20	2.96	2.81	2.70	2.61	2.55	2.49	2.45	2.38	2.31	2.23	2.19	2.15	2.10	2.06	2.01	1.96
18	4.41	3.55	3.16	2.93	2.77	2.66	2.58	2.51	2.46	2.41	2.34	2.27	2.19	2.15	2.11	2.06	2.02	1.97	1.92
19	4.38	3.52	3.13	2.90	2.74	2.63	2.54	2.48	2.42	2.38	2.31	2.23	2.16	2.11	2.07	2.03	1.98	1.93	1.88
20	4.35	3.49	3.10	2.87	2.71	2.60	2.51	2.45	2.39	2.35	2.28	2.20	2.12	2.08	2.04	1.99	1.95	1.90	1.84
21	4.32	3.47	3.07	2.84	2.68	2.57	2.49	2.42	2.37	2.32	2.25	2.18	2.10	2.05	2.01	1.96	1.92	1.87	1.81
22	4.30	3.44	3.05	2.82	2.66	2.55	2.46	2.40	2.34	2.30	2.23	2.15	2.07	2.03	1.98	1.94	1.89	1.84	1.78
23	4.28	3.42	3.03	2.80	2.64	2.53	2.44	2.37	2.32	2.27	2.20	2.13	2.05	2.01	1.96	1.91	1.86	1.81	1.76
24	4.26	3.40	3.01	2.78	2.62	2.51	2.42	2.36	2.30	2.25	2.18	2.11	2.03	1.98	1.94	1.89	1.84	1.79	1.73
25	4.24	3.39	2.99	2.76	2.60	2.49	2.40	2.34	2.28	2.24	2.16	2.09	2.01	1.96	1.92	1.87	1.82	1.77	1.71
26	4.23	3.37	2.98	2.74	2.59	2.47	2.39	2.32	2.27	2.22	2.15	2.07	1.99	1.95	1.90	1.85	1.80	1.75	1.69
27	4.21	3.35	2.96	2.73	2.57	2.46	2.37	2.31	2.25	2.20	2.13	2.06	1.97	1.93	1.88	1.84	1.79	1.73	1.67
28	4.20	3.34	2.95	2.71	2.56	2.45	2.36	2.29	2.24	2.19	2.12	2.04	1.96	1.91	1.87	1.82	1.77	1.71	1.65
29	4.18	3.33	2.93	2.70	2.55	2.43	2.35	2.28	2.22	2.18	2.10	2.03	1.94	1.90	1.85	1.81	1.75	1.70	1.64
30	4.17	3.32	2.92	2.69	2.53	2.42	2.33	2.27	2.21	2.16	2.09	2.01	1.93	1.89	1.84	1.79	1.74	1.68	1.62
40	4.08	3.23	2.84	2.61	2.45	2.34	2.25	2.18	2.12	2.08	2.00	1.92	1.84	1.79	1.74	1.69	1.64	1.58	1.51
60	4.00	3.15	2.76	2.53	2.37	2.25	2.17	2.10	2.04	1.99	1.92	1.84	1.75	1.70	1.65	1.59	1.53	1.47	1.39
120	3.92	3.07	2.68	2.45	2.29	2.17	2.09	2.02	1.96	1.91	1.83	1.75	1.66	1.61	1.55	1.50	1.43	1.35	1.25
∞	3.84	3.00	2.60	2.37	2.21	2.10	2.01	1.94	1.88	1.83	1.75	1.67	1.57	1.52	1.46	1.39	1.32	1.22	1.00

$F_{0.05}$

This table is taken from Table 18 of E S Pearson and H O Hartley (eds), *Biometrika Tables for Statisticians* Vol. 1, third edition (1966) by permission of the *Biometrika* Trustees.

Table 4(b)   Distribution of F—continued

The table entry is the critical value of F at 0.01 probability corresponding to the appropriate degrees of freedom for numerator (v_1) and denominator (v_2).

$F_{0.01}$

v_2 \ v_1	1	2	3	4	5	6	7	8	9	10	12	15	20	24	30	40	60	120	∞
1	4,052	4,999.5	5,403	5,625	5,764	5,859	5,928	5,981	6,022	6,056	6,106	6,157	6,209	6,235	6,261	6,287	6,313	6,339	6,366
2	98.50	99.00	99.17	99.25	99.30	99.33	99.36	99.37	99.39	99.40	99.42	99.43	99.45	99.46	99.47	99.47	99.48	99.49	99.50
3	34.12	30.82	29.46	28.71	28.24	27.91	27.67	27.49	27.35	27.23	27.05	26.87	26.69	26.60	26.50	26.41	26.32	26.22	26.13
4	21.20	18.00	16.69	15.98	15.52	15.21	14.98	14.80	14.66	14.55	14.37	14.20	14.02	13.93	13.84	13.75	13.65	13.56	13.46
5	16.26	13.27	12.06	11.39	10.97	10.67	10.46	10.29	10.16	10.05	9.89	9.72	9.55	9.47	9.38	9.29	9.20	9.11	9.02
6	13.75	10.92	9.78	9.15	8.75	8.47	8.26	8.10	7.98	7.87	7.72	7.56	7.40	7.31	7.23	7.14	7.06	6.97	6.88
7	12.25	9.55	8.45	7.85	7.46	7.19	6.99	6.84	6.72	6.62	6.47	6.31	6.16	6.07	5.99	5.91	5.82	5.74	5.65
8	11.26	8.65	7.59	7.01	6.63	6.37	6.18	6.03	5.91	5.81	5.67	5.52	5.36	5.28	5.20	5.12	5.03	4.95	4.86
9	10.56	8.02	6.99	6.42	6.06	5.80	5.61	5.47	5.35	5.26	5.11	4.96	4.81	4.73	4.65	4.57	4.48	4.40	4.31
10	10.04	7.56	6.55	5.99	5.64	5.39	5.20	5.06	4.94	4.85	4.71	4.56	4.41	4.33	4.25	4.17	4.08	4.00	3.91
11	9.65	7.21	6.22	5.67	5.32	5.07	4.89	4.74	4.63	4.54	4.40	4.25	4.10	4.02	3.94	3.86	3.78	3.69	3.60
12	9.33	6.93	5.95	5.41	5.06	4.82	4.64	4.50	4.39	4.30	4.16	4.01	3.86	3.78	3.70	3.62	3.54	3.45	3.36
13	9.07	6.70	5.74	5.21	4.86	4.62	4.44	4.30	4.19	4.10	3.96	3.82	3.66	3.59	3.51	3.43	3.34	3.25	3.17
14	8.86	6.51	5.56	5.04	4.69	4.46	4.28	4.14	4.03	3.94	3.80	3.66	3.51	3.43	3.35	3.27	3.18	3.09	3.00
15	8.68	6.36	5.42	4.89	4.56	4.32	4.14	4.00	3.89	3.80	3.67	3.52	3.37	3.29	3.21	3.13	3.05	2.96	2.87
16	8.53	6.23	5.29	4.77	4.44	4.20	4.03	3.89	3.78	3.69	3.55	3.41	3.26	3.18	3.10	3.02	2.93	2.84	2.75
17	8.40	6.11	5.18	4.67	4.34	4.10	3.93	3.79	3.68	3.59	3.46	3.31	3.16	3.08	3.00	2.92	2.83	2.75	2.65
18	8.29	6.01	5.09	4.58	4.25	4.01	3.84	3.71	3.60	3.51	3.37	3.23	3.08	3.00	2.92	2.84	2.75	2.66	2.57
19	8.18	5.93	5.01	4.50	4.17	3.94	3.77	3.63	3.52	3.43	3.30	3.15	3.00	2.92	2.84	2.76	2.67	2.58	2.49
20	8.10	5.85	4.94	4.43	4.10	3.87	3.70	3.56	3.46	3.37	3.23	3.09	2.94	2.86	2.78	2.69	2.61	2.52	2.42
21	8.02	5.78	4.87	4.37	4.04	3.81	3.64	3.51	3.40	3.31	3.17	3.03	2.88	2.80	2.72	2.64	2.55	2.46	2.36
22	7.95	5.72	4.82	4.31	3.99	3.76	3.59	3.45	3.35	3.26	3.12	2.98	2.83	2.75	2.67	2.58	2.50	2.40	2.31
23	7.88	5.66	4.76	4.26	3.94	3.71	3.54	3.41	3.30	3.21	3.07	2.93	2.78	2.70	2.62	2.54	2.45	2.35	2.26
24	7.82	5.61	4.72	4.22	3.90	3.67	3.50	3.36	3.26	3.17	3.03	2.89	2.74	2.66	2.58	2.49	2.40	2.31	2.21
25	7.77	5.57	4.68	4.18	3.85	3.63	3.46	3.32	3.22	3.13	2.99	2.85	2.70	2.62	2.54	2.45	2.36	2.27	2.17
26	7.72	5.53	4.64	4.14	3.82	3.59	3.42	3.29	3.18	3.09	2.96	2.81	2.66	2.58	2.50	2.42	2.33	2.23	2.13
27	7.68	5.49	4.60	4.11	3.78	3.56	3.39	3.26	3.15	3.06	2.93	2.78	2.63	2.55	2.47	2.38	2.29	2.20	2.10
28	7.64	5.45	4.57	4.07	3.75	3.53	3.36	3.23	3.12	3.03	2.90	2.75	2.60	2.52	2.44	2.35	2.26	2.17	2.06
29	7.60	5.42	4.54	4.04	3.73	3.50	3.33	3.20	3.09	3.00	2.87	2.73	2.57	2.49	2.41	2.33	2.23	2.14	2.03
30	7.56	5.39	4.51	4.02	3.70	3.47	3.30	3.17	3.07	2.98	2.84	2.70	2.55	2.47	2.39	2.30	2.21	2.11	2.01
40	7.31	5.18	4.31	3.83	3.51	3.29	3.12	2.99	2.89	2.80	2.66	2.52	2.37	2.29	2.20	2.11	2.02	1.92	1.80
60	7.08	4.98	4.13	3.65	3.34	3.12	2.95	2.82	2.72	2.63	2.50	2.35	2.20	2.12	2.03	1.94	1.84	1.73	1.60
120	6.85	4.79	3.95	3.48	3.17	2.96	2.79	2.66	2.56	2.47	2.34	2.19	2.03	1.95	1.86	1.76	1.66	1.53	1.38
∞	6.63	4.61	3.78	3.32	3.02	2.80	2.64	2.51	2.41	2.32	2.18	2.04	1.88	1.79	1.70	1.59	1.47	1.32	1.00

This table is taken from Table 18 of E S Pearson and H O Hartley (eds), *Biometrika Tables for Statisticians* Vol. 1, third edition (1966) by permission of the *Biometrika* Trustees.

Bibliography

Caulcott E (1973) *Significance Tests*. London: Routledge & Kegan Paul.

Croxton F E, Cowden D J and Klein S (1968) *Applied General Statistics*. London: Pitman.

Fisher R A and Yates F (1974 6th edn) *Statistical Tables for Biological, Agricultural and Medical Research*. Edinburgh: Oliver and Boyd.

Doll R and Hill A B (1950) 'Smoking and carcinoma of the lung' *British Medical Journal* **ii**, 739 included in Hill A B (1962) *Statistical Methods in Clinical and Preventive Medicine*. Edinburgh: Livingstone.

Molina E E (1947) *Poisson's Exponential Binomial Limit*. Princeton NJ: D Van Nostrand.

Pearson E S and Hartley H O (eds) (1966 3rd edn) *Biometrika Tables for Statisticians*. London: CUP.

Rand Corporation (1966) *A Million Random Digits with 100,000 Normal Deviates*. New York: Macmillan.

Siegel S and Castellan N J (1988 2nd edn) *Nonparametric statistics for the behavioural sciences*. New York: McGraw-Hill Kogakusha.

Walpole R E (1982 3rd edn) *Introduction to Statistics*. New York: Collier Macmillan.

A Little Practice—Answers

Chapter 2

1 (a) continuous (b) height, metres (c) lower class limits (ms) 1.55, 1.60, 1.65, 1.70, 1.75, 1.80, 1.85; upper class limits (ms) 1.59, 1.64, 1.69, 1.74, 1.79, 1.84, 1.89 (d) class boundaries (ms) 1.545, 1.595, 1.645, 1.695, 1.745, 1.795, 1.845, 1.895 (e) midpoints (ms) 1.57, 1.62, 1.67, 1.72, 1.77, 1.82, 1.87 (f) yes, 0.05 ms (5 cms). **2** (a) discrete (b) occupied beds, beds (c) lower class limits (beds) 10, 16, 18, 20, 22, 24; upper class limits (beds) 15, 17, 19, 21, 23, 25 (d) class boundaries (beds) 9.5, 15.5, 17.5, 19.5, 21.5, 23.5, 25.5 (e) class midpoints (beds) 12.5, 16.5, 18.5, 20.5, 22.5, 24.5 (f) no; first class interval is 6 beds, remainder 2 beds. **3** (a) discrete (b) out-patient visits, visits (c) lower class limits (visits) 1, 2, 3, 4, 5, 6; upper class limits (visits) 1, 2, 3, 4, 5, 8 (d) class boundaries (visits) 0.5, 1.5, 2.5, 3.5, 4.5, 5.5, 8.5 (e) class midpoints (visits) 1, 2, 3, 4, 5, 7 (f) no; highest class has interval of 3 visits, the others 1 visit.

Chapter 4

1 (a) 3.8, 16.2, 37.1, 28.3, 9.5, 4.3, 0.7 (b) 4, 16, 37, 28, 10, 4, 1. **2** As the total being turned into percentages (30) is very small, percentages are expressed as whole numbers. 7, 10, 17, 23, 27, 17 [Percentages do not always add to 100 because of rounding.]. **3** 2.88, 2.58, 2.45, 3.2, 3.57, 3.11, 2.6, 2.08, 2.27, 2.44. **4** 87, 83, 83, 89, 86, 80, 91, 88, 93, 87.

Chapter 5

First decile for hospital dental staff (see section 9):

$$25 + \frac{123.5}{398} \times 5 = 26.6 \text{ years}$$

1 (a) 6 days (b) 5 days. **2** Both measures are 1.69 ms. **3** The heights read off from the ogive *approximate* to (a) 1.66 ms, 1.73 ms (b) 1.65 ms, 1.74 ms (c) 1.62 ms, 1.77 ms. **4** Using midpoints (years) 25, 37.5, 52.5 and 65 (a) 49.9 years (b) 51.5 years (c) 40.8 years, 60.3 years.

Chapter 6

1 0.0575 ms (5.75 cms).   **2** 3.6 visits, 1.48 visits.   **3** Using the midpoints as for calculating the mean [Chapter 5 answer to question 4 above] 12.2 years.   **4** Using 12 days as the midpoint for the open-ended class, 5.42 days, 1.80 days.

Chapter 7

1 (a) 0.6 (b) 0.3 (c) 0.4.   **2** (a) 0.09 (b) 0.01 (c) 0.12.   **3** (a) 0.001 (b) 0.216 (c) 0.108.

Chapter 8

Theoretical answers **1** (a) 2 heads (b) 1 heads. **2** (a) 5 heads (b) 1.58 heads.

Chapter 10

1 $se_{\bar{x}}$ = £0.11, 95% c.l. £30.28 to £30.72, 99% c.l. £30.22 to £30.78. **2** $se_{\bar{x}}$ = 0.085 days, 95% c.l. 4.73 to 5.07 days.   **3** $se_{\bar{x}}$ = 0.45 days, 99.9% c.l. 43.9 to 46.9 days.   **4** se_p = 2.30%, 95% c.l. 70.5% to 79.5% **5** se_p = 3.96%, 99% c.l. 51.8% to 72.2%.   **6** p = 71.85%, se_p = 3.87%, 95% c.l. 64.3% to 79.4%.

Chapter 12

1 $se_{\bar{x}}$ = 0.1645 years, z = 4.26.   **2** $se_{\bar{x}}$ = 0.6188 days, z = −7.27. **3** se_p = 2.21%, z = −1.04.   **4** p = 71.90%, se_p = 3.63%, z = −2.23. **5** $se_{\bar{x}_1 - \bar{x}_2}$ = 30.63 patients, z = 1.66.   **6** $se_{\bar{x}_1 - \bar{x}_2}$ = 0.380 days, z = 1.84. **7** $se_{p_1 - p_2}$ = 5.73%, z = −0.35.   **8** p_1 = 85.45%, p_2 = 76.67%, $se_{p_1 - p_2}$ = 3.13%, z = 2.81.

Chapter 13

1 4 degrees of freedom, χ^2 = 24.868, $p < 0.001$ Scheme A has more satisfied maternity patients ('very' and 'fairly' satisfied taken together) and fewer than expected who were dissatisfied.   **2** 4 degrees of freedom, χ^2 = 7.923, $0.10 < p < 0.05$. An indeterminate result in that the Null Hypothesis cannot be rejected. It suggests Regime B might be superior but more information is required.   **3** 5 degrees of freedom, χ^2 = 97.606, $p < 0.001$. Very strong association. Professional men, employers and managers are less likely than expected to have consulted their general practitioner; markedly more unskilled manual workers than expected had consulted their general practitioners.   **4** 2 degrees of freedom, χ^2 = 2.226, $p < 0.30$. Accept the Null Hypothesis. There is no statistical evidence that one treatment is superior to the other.

Chapter 14

1 Sample means (hours) $x_1 = 3.5$, $x_2 = 3.1$, $x_3 = 3.8$; sample variances $s_1^2 = 0.75$, $s_2^2 = 0.54$, $s_3^2 = 0.51$; $s_b^2 = 1.233$, $s_w^2 = 0.6$, $F = 2.06$. Degrees of freedom for numerator 2, for denominator 27, $F_{0.05} = 3.35$. The Null Hypothesis is not rejected; the differences between the analgesics in their effectiveness could be due to sampling error.   **2** Sample means (courses of treatment) $x_1 = 3.5$, $x_2 = 5$, $x_3 = 6$; $s_1^2 = 3$, $s_2^2 = 3$, $s_3^2 = 2$; $s_b^2 = 12.667$, $s_w^2 = 2.667$, $F = 4.75$. Degrees of freedom for numerator 2, for denominator 21, $F_{0.05} = 3.47$, $F_{0.01} = 5.78$. The Null Hypothesis is rejected at 0.05 probability but not at 0.01 probability; the data suggests that treatment A may be more effective than treatments B or C.

Chapter 16

1 $y = 6.54 + 0.778x$ (a)   38   patients   (b)   43   patients.   **2**   (b) $y = 19.53 - 0.2x$ (c) 0.2% decline between successive intakes (d) 16.1, 15.5. Possibly   since the rate of decline between intakes is fairly low, but the rate of decline must eventually tail off.   **3** $r = 0.88$ indicating a strong association. **4** (b) $r = 0.85$, $r' = 0.90$ (c) The relationship is curvilinear (see scatter diagram) so that the rank correlation coefficient is a better measure of a quite close agreement between the assessors.

Note. The precise results of computations depend on the detailed accuracy of the actual process. If computations are carried out with the full accuracy of a pocket calculator (up to eight significant figures), or using a statistical package on a computer, the end results will be marginally different from the answers that would have been obtained from reasonable rounding at different stages during the process of computation. Different ways of handling data can also produce slight variations between answers achieved through reasonable alternative assumptions.

Do not be surprised if your results from A Little Practice are marginally different from the answers given here. What matters is that orders of magnitude should be correct, that you should be able to process data to obtain a reasonable result. Do not worry about very small differences.

Index